HYPERTENSION
recent advances and research

Proceedings of the International Symposium of Sorrento on «Recent advances in hypertension research» (Sorrento, October 18-20, 1980)

Editors:
M. Condorelli, A. Zanchetti

Scientific Committee:
G. Brevetti, M. Chiariello
Institute of Medical Pathology,
New Polyclinic, 80131 Naples, Italy

Published with the assistance of a grant made by Glaxo S.p.A., Verona (Italy)

HYPERTENSION

recent advances and research

Edited by
Mario Condorelli
Institute of Medical Pathology, University of Naples, Italy
Alberto Zanchetti
Institute of Cardiovascular Research, University of Milan, Italy

A Cortina Medical Publication

cortina international · verona

distributed by

Raven Press/New York

Cortina International · Verona
a branch of
Edizioni Libreria Cortina Verona S.r.l.
Via C. Cattaneo, 8 - 37121 Verona (Italy)
Tel. 045/38821 - 594818
Telex 431107 CORTIN I

© Copyright 1982
ISBN 88-85037-38-0

Printed in Italy by Edizioni Libreria Cortina Verona
Via C. Cattaneo 8 - 37121 Verona (Italy)

Contributors

AGABITI-ROSEI, E.
Department V of Clinical Medicine, University of Milan, Civic Hospitals, EULO, Brescia, Italy

ALICANDRI, C.
Department V of Clinical Medicine, University of Milan, Civic Hospitals, EULO, Brescia, Italy

AMBROSIONI, E.
Department of Cardiology and Department of Clinical Pharmacology, University of Bologna, Italy

ANDREOZZI, G.M.
2nd Institute of Special Pathological Medicine and Clinical Methodology, University of Catania, Italy

ANGELINO, P.F.
Department of Cardiology, St. John the Baptist's Hospital, Turin, Italy

BESCHI, M.
Department V of Clinical Medicine, University of Milan, Civic Hospitals, EULO, Brescia, Italy

BOMPIANI, G.D.
3rd Institute of General Clinical and Therapeutic Medicine, University of Palermo, Italy

BONI, E.
Department V of Clinical Medicine, University of Milan, Civic Hospitals, EULO, Brescia, Italy

BOSCIA, F.
Department of Diseases of the Cardiovascular Apparatus, University of Bari, Italy

BREVETTI, G.
Institute of Medical Pathology, 2nd School of Medicine, Naples, Italy

BURAGLIO, M.
Department of Cardiology, St. John the Baptist's Hospital, Turin, Italy

CARAVELLI, M.
Institute of General Clinical and Therapeutic Medicine, University of Messina, Italy

CASTELLANO, M.
Department V of Clinical Medicine, University of Milan, Civic Hospital, EULO, Brescia, Italy

CERASOLA, G.A.
3rd Institute of General Clinical and Therapeutic Medicine, University of Palermo, Italy

CHERCHI, A.
Department of Cardiovascular Pathology, University of Cagliari, Italy

CHIARIELLO, M.
Institute of Medical Pathology, 2nd School of Medicine, Naples, Italy

CHIATTO, M.
Department of Cadiology, Cosenza, Civic Hospital, Italy

CHIDDO, A.
Department of Diseases of the Cardiovascular Apparatus, University of Bari, Italy

CONDORELLI, M.
Institute of Medical Pathology, 2nd School of Medicine, Naples, Italy

CONSOLO, F.
Institute of General Clinical and Therapeutic Medicine, University of Messina, Italy

COSTA, F.V.
Department of Cardiology and Department of Clinical Pharmacology, University of Bologna, Italy

CURIA, F.
Department of Cardiology, Cosenza, Civic Hospital, Italy

DAVÌ, G.
Institute of Clinical Medicine and Medical Therapy of University of Palermo, Italy

DONATELLI, M.
3rd Institute of General Clinical and Therapeutic Medicine, University of Palermo, Italy

FARIELLO, F.
Department V of Clinical Medicine, University of Milan, Civic Hospital, EULO, Brescia, Italy

FAZIO, M.
Institute of Clinical Medicine and Medical Therapy of University of Palermo, Italy

FRANCHINI, G.
Department of Diseases of the Cardiovascular Apparatus, University of Bari, Italy

GAGLIONE, A.
Department of Diseases of the Cardiovascular Apparatus, University of Bari, Italy

GENOVESE, A.
Institute of Medical Pathology, 2nd School of Medicine, Naples, Italy

KOCH, G.
Department of Clinical Physiology, Central Hospital, Karlskrona, Sweden and Department of Physiology, Free University of Berlin, West Germany

LAVECCHIA, G.
Institute of Medical Pathology, University of Naples, Italy

LAVEZZARO, G.C.
Department of Cardiology, St. John the Baptist's Hospital, Turin, Italy

LICATA, G.
Institute of Medical Pathology «R», University of Palermo, Italy

LUZZA, G.
Institute of General Clinical and Therapeutic Medicine, University of Messina, Italy

MAGNANI, B.
Department of Cardiology and Department of Clinical Pharmacology, University of Bologna, Italy

MASTRANGELO, D.
Department of Diseases of the Cardiovascular Apparatus, University of Bari, Italy

MONTEBUGNOLI, L.
Department of Cardiology and Department of Clinical Pharmacology, University of Bologna, Italy

MONTINI, E.
Department V of Clinical Medicine, University of Milan, Civic Hospital, EULO, Brescia, Italy

MORICI, M.L.
3rd Institute of General Clinical and Therapeutic Medicine, University of Palermo, Italy

MUIESAN, G.
Department V of Clinical Medicine, University of Milan, Civic Hospital, EULO, Brescia, Italy

MUIESAN M.L.
Department V of Clinical Medicine, University of Milan, Civic Hospital, EULO, Brescia, Italy

NOVO, S.
Institute of Clinical Medicine and Medical Therapy of University of Palermo, Italy

PINTO, A.
Institute of Clinical Medicine and Medical Therapy of University of Palermo, Italy

PITRONE, F.
Institute of General Clinical and Therapeutic Medicine, University of Messina, Italy

PLASTINA, F.
Department of Cardiology, Cosenza, Civic Hospital, Italy

PUSTORINO, S.
Institute of General Clinical and Therapeutic Medicine University, of Messina, Italy

QUAGLIARA, D.
Department of Diseases of the Cardiovascular Apparatus, University of Bari, Italy

RENGO, F.
Institute of Medical Pathology, 2nd Medical School, University of Naples, Italy

RICHARDS, D.A
Glaxo Group Research Ltd., Ware, Hertfordshire, Great Britain

RIZZON, P.
Department of Diseases of the Cardiovascular Apparatus, University of Bari, Italy

ROMANELLI, G.
Department V of Clinical Medicine, University of Milan, Civic Hospital, EULO, Brescia, Italy

RUSSO, A.
Institute of General Clinical and Therapeutic Medicine, University of Messina, Italy

SALCEDO, E.A.
Cleveland Clinic Foundation, Cleveland, U.S.A.

SALERNO, L.
Institute of Medical Pathology «R», University of Palermo, Italy

SIGNORELLI, S.
2nd Institute of Special Pathological Medicine and Clinical Methodology, University of Catania, Italy

SORRENTINO, F.
2nd Institute of Special Pathological Medicine and Clinical Methodology, University of Catania, Italy

STRANO, A.
Institute of Clinical Medicine and Medical Therapy of University of Palermo, C.N.R.-Preventive Medicine Project, Hypertension Sub-project, University of Palermo, Italy

TARTAGNI, F.
Department of Cardiology and Department of Clinical Pharmacology, University of Bologna, Italy

VENNERI, N.
Department of Cardiology, Cosenza, Civic Hospital, Italy

VERRIENTI, S.
Institute of Medical Pathology, University of Naples, Italy

VIGORITO, G.
Institute of Medical Pathology, University of Naples, Italy

ZANCHETTI, A.
Institute of Cardiovascular Research, University of Milan, Italy

Contents

HYPERTENSION
recent advances and research

Hypertension, recent advances and research
edited by M. Condorelli, A. Zanchetti
Cortina International, Verona 1982

Research on the effects of Labetalol treatment on PRA and plasma aldosterone in primary hypertension

F. CONSOLO, A. RUSSO, F. PITRONE, S. PUSTORINO, G. LUZZA, M. CARAVELLI

Institute of General Clinical and Therapeutic Medicine, University of Messina

Key words. Labetalol; Plasma Renin Activity; Plasma Aldosterone; Primary Hypertension; Electrolyte Balance; Kidney Damage.

Summary. An investigation has been made into the behaviour of plasma renin activity and plasma aldosterone levels in hypertensive patients on Labetalol treatment, concomitantly with the effects on blood pressure, heart rate and electrolyte balance.

The case study comprised 25 subjects (9 males and 16 females ranging in age from 21 to 79 years with an average age of 58 years) suffering from primary hypertension, 6 of whom with kidney damage, and on a standard hospital diet.

The Labetalol treatment was given in the form of a 400 mg. dose per day in two oral administrations daily. The PRA assay data on day six revealed a significant reduction in PRA in 52% of cases, while no variation was observed in the other 48%. The plasma aldosterone assay on day six also revealed no significant variations in plasma aldosterone values as compared to basal values and this paralleled the non-significance of the modest variations in hydro-electrolytic balance.

The results demonstrate that in hypertensive subjects Labetalol treatment at the dose of 400 mg. per day brings about a reduction in PRA which is independent of the existence of high basal PRA values, but is closely related to the anti-hypertensive effect induced by the drug.

The study of the changes brought about by the blockade of the beta-adrenoceptors on the renin-angiotensin-aldosterone system in arterial hypertension has proved to be a highly fertile field of research supplying useful results for understanding the mechanisms of the anti-hypertensive action of the beta-blockers. It has also demonstrated its validity as a method of deeper pathophysiological and pathogenetic analysis of arterial hypertensive conditions.

The effects of a combined alpha- and beta-receptor blockade on renin secretion and on the plasma levels of aldosterone in arterial hypertension have been the subject of recent experimental and clinical studies. This line of research received a stimulus with the creation of Labetalol, a drug whose pharmacological profile is characterized by a combined alpha- and beta-blocking action [1-6], which motivated clinical experimentation and later therapeutic use of the drug for the treatment of arterial hypertension.

It is a known fact that beta-blocking drugs decrease plasma renin levels and that this inhibiting action is explained by the non-activation of adenyl cyclase and, consequently, the non-increase in cyclic-AMP formation as a result of the adrenergic effector [7, 8].

At the same time, the alpha-blocking action has the effect of stimulating the secretion of renin both "in vivo" and "in vitro", forming a model activator of renin incretion independent of the mediated vasodilatory effects and the consequent adrenoceptor haemodynamic reflex reactions. This effect is explained by the increased availability of norepinephrine for the beta-blocking activation of adenyl cyclase and the increase in cyclic-AMP formation [9].

With regard to the combined alpha- and beta-blockade in man, the intravenous administration of Labetalol has been seen to bring about a rapid reduction in PRA.

This reduction is already apparent (Agabiti-Rosei et al. of the Muiesan group) as little as 30 minutes after acute administration of the drug [10].

The authors describe it as being of moderate proportions and underline its significant correlation with high basal levels of PRA and plasma catecholamines.

In treatment on the basis of the medium-term oral administration of increasing doses of Labetalol, the reduction in PRA proved to be directly related to the basal levels of the enzyme and appeared to decline on administration of medium-high oral doses, as opposed to the progressive trend recorded for low and medium-low doses of Labetalol [11].

No correlation was observed between the decrease in PRA and the anti-hypertensive effects of Labetalol. The aim of the study was to evaluate the effects produced by oral treatment with Labetalol on the renin-angiotensin-aldosterone system, along with its BP and HR restraining capability and its influence on sodium and potassium balance, in patients suffering from primary hypertension.

Study protocol

The 25 patients participating in the trial, 9 males and 16 females aged between 21 and 79 years (M + SD 58 ± 12.5) were hypertensives of WHO Classes 1 (14), 2 (9) and 3 (2), six of whom were suffering from renal impairment (Table I).

All were admitted to hospital one week before the commencement of the study and kept on a standard diet of 80 mEq/day of sodium and potassium.

Treatment with Labetalol was initiated after a 14-day wash-out and maintained at a dosage of 400 mg/day in two oral administrations daily.

Twelve patients who showed no anti-hypertensive effects after 5 days were administered a single 40 mg intravenous dose of Furosemide in the morning on days 6, 7 and 8.

The study parameters consisted in the determination of: PRA in the supine and upright

Table I. *Patients participating in the trial (25).*

SEX	16		9	
AGE RANGE = 21-79 (M=58)	55 YEARS 32% (8)		55 YEARS 68% (17)	
DURATION OF HYPERTENSION	5 YEARS 44% (11)		5 YEARS 56% (14)	
DEGREE OF HYPERTENSION	SLIGHT 56% (14)	MODERATE 36% (9)		SEVERE 8% (2)
RENAL FUNCTION	WITH RENAL IMPAIRMENT 24% (6)		WITHOUT RENAL IMPAIRMENT 76% (19)	
NATRIURESIS	WITH SODIUM RETENTION 56% (14)		WITHOUT SODIUM RETENTION 44% (11)	
PRA	NORMAL 36% (9)	HIGH 4% (1		LOW 60% (15)

positions (associated with muscular activity), plasma aldosterone levels at 8 a.m. and 6 p.m., plasma Na+ and plasma K+ values, and the quantities of sodium and potassium excreted daily.

Patients' BP was measured daily, in both the supine and upright positions, using a conventional sphygmomanometer, and at the same time heart rate was recorded. The measurements were repeated 4 times a day: at 8 a.m., 12 noon, 4 p.m. and 8 p.m.

PRA and plasma aldosterone were assessed by a radioimmuno-assay using sensitized test tubes provided in kits by CEA-CIS-SORIN.

Serum and urine potassium and sodium levels were determined using a flame spectro-photometer.

The quantitative analysis of the study parameters was carried out on the deltas, i.e. on the differences between the pre- and post-treatment values, applying Student's "t" test for paired data, calculated in terms of the ratio of the mean delta values to the standard deviations so as to check out the significance of the differences between pre- and post-treatment.

The delta values were examined by means of variance analysis, isolating parellelisms between PRA and BP to check out any possibile correlations between changes observed during treatment.

The PRA assays were effected before treatment, after 14 days' wash-out, on 2 consecutive days, with the calculation of the mean values obtained after 5 days of treatment in all patients and - in the case of the 12 patients who were given 3 consecutive daily i.v. doses of Furosemide - on the 9th day of treatment.

Plasma aldosterone values were determined parally prior to treatment, on 2 consecutive days, and repeated every day throughout the therapy. Serum sodium and potassium levels and the urinary excretion of the same were determined simultaneously along with the aldosterone assays on 2 consecutive days before treatment began and every day throughout the trial period.

Basal PRA values in the supine and upright positions were found to be low in 16 patients, normal in 8 and high in 1.

Basal plasma aldosterone values were with-

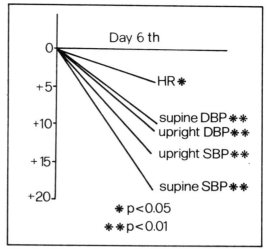

Fig. 1. Effects of Labetalol (400 mg/day) on BP and HR in 25 primary hypertension subjects.

in the normal range, both at 8 a.m. and at 6 p.m., in all patients except one, who - along with high PRA - had plasma aldosterone values varying between 553 Pg/ml (8 a.m.) and 853 Pg/ml (6 p.m.).

The sodium balance was normal in 11 patients and positive in 14. None of the patients showed any sign of increased potassemia.

As illustrated in Fig. 1, the quantitative analysis of the deltas after 5 days of oral treatment with Labetalol revealed a highly significant reduction - statistically speaking - in systolic and diastolic BP in both the supine and upright positions ($P < 0.01$ - SBP supine MD 18.8 - DBP supine MD 10 - SBP upright MD 14.2 - DBP upright MD 11), and a moderate reduction in heart rate (MD 3.68) of low statistical significance ($P < 0.05$).

At the clinical level, the anti-hypertensive effect was apparent in 52% of the patients whilst blood pressure variations in the other 48% were only moderate or negligible.

In those who responded to the treatment, systolic and diastolic BP values registered a gradual reduction, usually beginning within 48 hours and reaching maximum effect on the 5th day of therapy (Table II).

On the contrary, in those patients not responding to the treatment, not only were systolic and diastolic BP variations of modest

Table II. *BP and HR behaviour in 5 days treatment with Labetalol in the responsive subjects.*

DAY OF TREATMENT		1°	2°	3°	4°	5°
SBP	L	7.69	18.8	26.5	26.9	35
	SD	6.9	12.6	17.6	12.8	10.2
		★★	★★	★★	★★	★★
DBP	L	5.0	5.0	13.4	14.6	18.4
	SD	6.4	6.4	10.4	5.5	7.2
		★	★	★★	★★	★★
HR	L	1.77	3.0	3.53	4.0	4.15
	SD	1.92	3.36	4.7	6.78	6.7
		★★	★★	★	n.s.	★

★ $P < 0.05$
★★ $P < 0.01$

Table III. *Responsive (N. = 13).*

WITH RENAL IMPAIRMENT 30.7% (n=4)		WITHOUT RENAL IMPAIRMENT 69.3% (n=9)
WITH SODIUM RETENTION 53.8% (n=7)		WITHOUT SODIUM RETENTION 46.2% (n=6)
MORE THAN 55 YEARS OLD 76.9% (n=10)		LESS THAN 55 YEARS OLD 23.1% (n=3)
HYPERTENSIVE FOR MORE THAN 5 YEARS 53.8% (n=7)		HYPERTENSIVE FOR LESS THAN 5 YEARS 46.2% (n=6)
NORMAL PRA 46.2% (n=6)	LOW PRA 53.8% (n=7)	HIGH PRA 0% (n=0)

proportions (10 mmHg and 5 mmHg respectively), but they were also retarded, usually noted around the 4th day of treatment.

The quantitative analysis of the deltas for the BP and HR parameters and Student's "t" highlight, in the responsive patients, the statistical significance of the reduction in HR and the low value of the corresponding mean difference (MD = 4.1).

In terms of general responsiveness, Labetalol was observed to have an anti-hypertensive action in 66% of the patients with renal impairment and in 47% of those with normal renal function. In relation to the duration of the hypertensive condition, an anti-hypertensive effect was found in 63% of the patients suffering from the disease for more than 5 years and in only 35% of those whose condition was of more recent date.

Finally, no discriminatory anti-hypertensive effect was found in relation to the patient's age or to the positivity or otherwise of the sodium balance.

If the responsive patients are considered in relation to their renal condition, sodium retention, age, duration of hypertension and PRA, it is apparent that the anti-hypertensive effect was greater in patients with no renal impairment (69.3%), in patients with sodium retention (53.8%), in those over the age of 55 (76.9%), in those hypertensive for more than 5 years (53.8%) and in patients with low PRA (53.8%) (Table III).

Effects on PRA and plasma aldosterone

The effects of oral treatment with Labetalol on the basal and maximal PRA levels and on

4

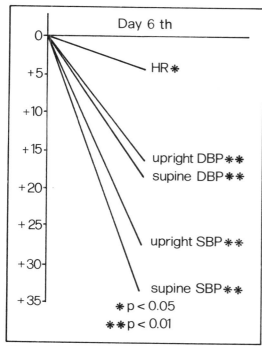

Fig. 2. Effects of Labetalol (400 mg/day) on BP and HR in 13 subjects responsive to treatment.

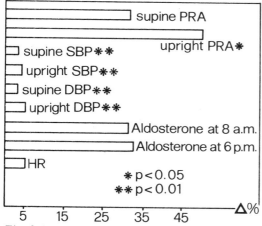

Fig. 3. Mean percentage deviations found on the 6th day of treatment with Labetalol (400 mg/day).

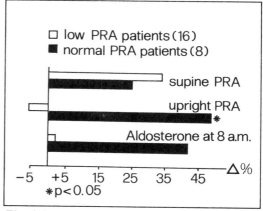

Fig. 4. Mean percentage differences of basal and maximal PRA and of aldesteronemia in normal and low-PRA patients observed after 5 days' treatment with Labetalol.

sal PRA and plasma aldosterone did not decrease significantly, but there was a statistically significant reduction in BP. Only maximal PRA variations were of moderate statistical importance ($P < 0.05$).

In relation to basal PRA and plasma aldosterone levels (Fig. 4), the mean percentage differences in the decreasing effect are significant only for maximal PRA, but of little statistical importance in normal-PRA subjects and of no importance in low-PRA subjects.

There was no difference in the decrease in basal and maximal PRA and plasma aldosterone levels in those patients who had an antihypertensive response.

Fig. 5 illustrates that the mean differences in the PRA and plasma aldosterone values of the

plasma aldosterone are illustrated in Fig. 3 which shows the mean percentage differences found on the 5th day of treatment in all patients participating in the trial.

After 5 days of treatment, both PRA and plasma aldosterone values had decreased. Ba-

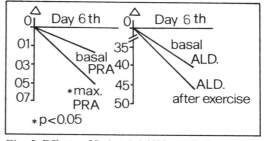

Fig. 5. Effects of Labetalol (400 mg/day) on PRA and plasma aldosterone in 13 responsive subjects.

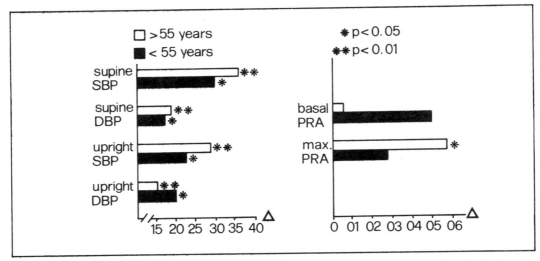

Fig. 6. Effects of Labetalol (400 mg/day) on BP and PRA in 13 responsive patients, in relation to age.

responsive patients increased as compared to those found in the patients as a whole and that the decrease in PRA is significant only in the maximal case, whilst plasma aldosterone undergoes no significant change at all.

The data shown demonstrate quite clearly that after 5 days' treatment with Labetalol (400 mg/day), the basal PRA and plasma aldosterone levels undergo a daily reduction of no great significance and that the maximal PRA decrease is of slight statistical importance; these data contrast strongly with the statistically highly significant reduction in systolic and diastolic BP in both the supine and upright positions.

The PRA and plasma aldosterone variations were assessed in relation to the age of the patient, the duration of the hypertension and the presence or otherwise of sodium retention or renal impairment.

Fig. 6 shows that there is a relationship, albeit of only slight importance, between the patient's age and the variations in the decrease in maximal PRA ($P < 0.05$), the mean differences being greater only in patients over 55 years of age.

As illustrated in Fig. 7, no statistical significance may be attributed to variations in basal and maximal PRA as far as the duration of

the hypertensive condition is concerned. The same was observed as regards the presence or absence of sodium retention (Fig. 8) and renal impairment (Fig. 9).

The plasma Na + and plasma K + values, determined by means of daily assays throughout the entire observation period, underwent extremely modest and insignificant increases, whilst urinary excretion of sodium and potassium remained virtually unchanged (Table IV). The responsive behaviour of the sodium and potassium balance was found to be the same in patients with pre-treatment sodium retention as in those without.

By analyzing the interrelationships between the parameters studied it was possibile to establish a correlation between decreasing systolic BP and maximal PRA variations only in those hypertensive patients who responded to the therapy with a striking reduction in BP values (Fig. 10).

No other correlation was observed between any of the other study parameters.

Those patients who failed to respond to oral treatment with Labetalol alone, and who were also given intravenous administrations of Furosemide in a single daily dose of 40 mg (Fig. 11), on the 9th day displayed a reduction in systolic BP in both the supine and upright

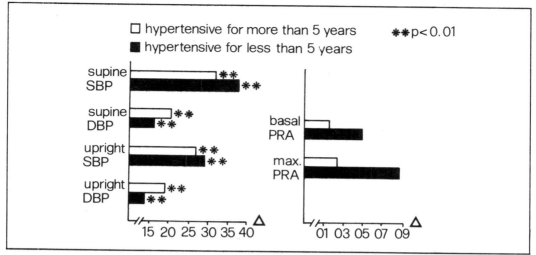

Fig. 7. Effects of Labetalol (400 mg/day) on BP and PRA in 13 responsive subjects, in relation to the duration of the hypertension.

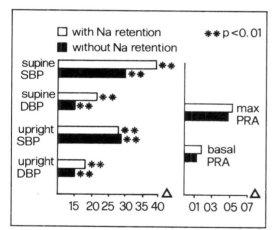

Fig. 8. Effects of Labetalol (400 mg/day) on BP and PRA in 13 responsive patients, in relation to the presence or otherwise of sodium retention.

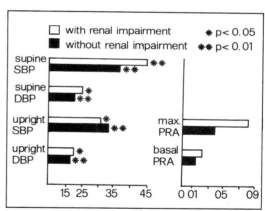

Fig. 9. Effects of Labetalol (400 mg/day) on BP and PRA in 13 responsive patients, in relation to the presence or otherwise of renal impairment.

Table IV. *Effects of oral treatment with Labetalol (400 mg/day) on the Sodium and Potassium balance in 25 subjects with primary hypertension.*

Na (P)	$\Delta = -0.88$ SD = 3.55 n.s.	Na (U)	$\Delta = -3.96$ SD = 18.3 n.s.
K (P)	$\Delta = -0.116$ SD = 0.4 n.s.	K (U)	$\Delta = -0.04$ SD = 0.53 n.s.

7

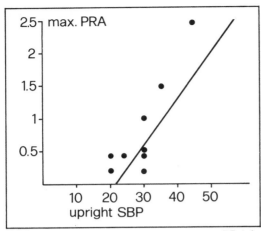

Fig. 10. Correlation between SBP and max. PRA in 13 patients responsive to treatment with Labetalol. $r = 0.7, P < 0.01$.

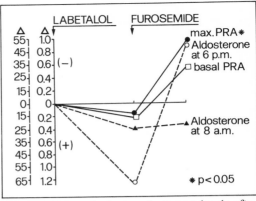

Fig. 12. PRA and plasma adosterone levels after treatment with Labetalol and with Labetalol + furosemide in 12 patients not responsive to single-drug treatment with Labetalol.

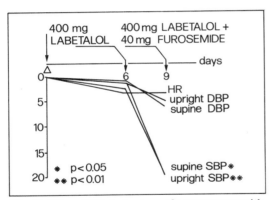

Fig. 11. BP and HR behaviour after treatment with Labetalol and with Labetalol + furosemide in 12 patients not responsive to single-drug treatment with Labetalol.

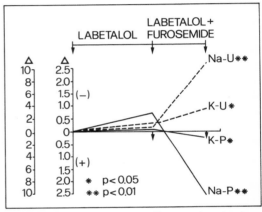

Fig. 13. Effects on the sodium and potassium balance of treatment with Labetalol and with Labetalol + furosemide in 12 patients not responsive to single-drug treatment.

positions, of greater statistical significance in the latter case at the same time as a noticeable decrease in diastolic BP in both positions.

Heart rate underwent no alteration.

Fig. 12 shows the PRA and plasma aldosterone variations in these patients on the 9th day after combined therapy with Labetalol and Furosemide. It can be observed that maximal PRA increased; both parameters are of moderate statistical importance (P 0.05). Basal PRA increase, however, is insignificant, whilst the morning plasma aldosterone levels are unchanged.

Fig. 13 shows the variations found on the 9th day, after combined Labetalol-Furosemide treatment, in relation to the serum levels of sodium and potassium and the urinary excretion of these two electrolytes. It is noted that, by the 9th day, serum sodium and potassium values have decreased considerably, whereas the urinary excretion levels of the two electrolytes have increased significantly.

The above data prove that the association of Furosemide and oral Labetalol, promotes the expected anti-hypertensive effect, corresponding variations in the urinary excretion of sodium and potassium and their serum levels, and consistent variations in PRA and plasma aldosterone levels.

Nevertheless, a statistical evaluation of the modifications observed in PRA and plasma aldosterone reveals a non-significant increase in basal PRA, a maximal PRA increase of modest significance and a differential behaviour on the part of plasma aldosterone levels, as characterized by an increase of low significance in evening levels of the hormone and no morning variation in plasma aldosterone.

These data seem to suggest a possible interference on the part of oral Labetalol treatment in the incremental variations induced by Furosemide in the renin-angiotensin-aldosterone system.

To check out this possibility, a test was carried out on 3 hypertensive patients, not included in the study, who were already hospitalized and had been on therapeutic anti-hypertensive wash-out for 14 days, with a standard diet of 80 mEq of sodium and potassium per day. The experimental procedure adopted was the following:
- determination of basal and maximal PRA on 2 consecutive days;
- daily intravenous injection every morning of 40 mg of Furosemide for 3 days;
- determination on day 4 of basal and maximal PRA;
- 5 days of wash-out;
- a second determination of PRA on 2 consecutive days;
- combined therapy with Labetalol (400 mg/day) and Furosemide (40 mg/day, i.v., in the morning) for 3 consecutive days;
- determination of PRA on day 4;
- 5 days of wash-out;
- resumption of treatment with Labetalol (400 mg/day);
- determination of PRA on day 6.

The results of this experiment are shown in Fig. 14. It can be seen that after 3 days of Furosemide basal and maximal PRA revealed percentage increases of 50% and 60% respectively.

When treatment with Furosemide is combined with the oral administration of Labetalol, the percentage increases for both basal and

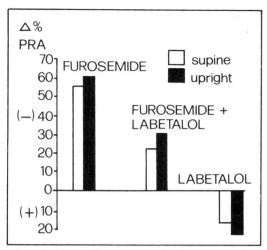

Fig. 14. PRA after treatment with furosemide, furosemide + Labetalol and Labetalol in 3 patients with primary hypertension.

maximal PRA are halved, as compared to those produced by treatment with Furosemide alone, whereas Labetalol alone has a decreasing effect of not more that 20% on maximal PRA and even less on basal PRA.

Discussion

With specific reference to the aims of this study, i.e. the examination of the effects of oral treatment with Labetalol at the standard dose of 400 mg/day on the responsive behaviour of the renin-angiotensin-aldosterone system in patients with primary hypertension, the first important observation to be made is that the oral administration of Labetalol at the above dose has a statistically significant anti-hypertensive effect.

Consequently, our dosage and the method of administration employed are sufficient to bring about the anti-hypertensive effect expected of this drug.

The second important element consists in the modifications in the renin-angiontensin-aldosterone system found after 5 days' treatment with Labetalol as revealed by the decrease (of little significance) only in the case of maximal PRA, and the insignificance of the decremental variations in plasma aldosterone.

The two phenomena, i.e. the reduction in

blood pressure and the reduction in maximal PRA, appear to have developed side by side, suggesting an interrelationship which would seem to find confirmation in the highly significant correlation between the decremental variations in maximal PRA and the reduction in systolic BP observed in patients whose antihypertensive response to the drug was clinically very evident.

Within the admittedly limited context of this small group of hypertensives, the above-mentioned correlations would tend to bear out the hypothesis of a possible interrelationship between these two effects.

In point of fact, the variations produced by oral treatment with Labetalol in the renin-angiotensin-aldosterone system show once again the same patterns of beta-blockade interference as are caused by other beta-receptor blockers and pose the same problems of interpretation, not so much with regard to the interference mechanism itself as with regard to the significance they assume in relation to the renin-inhibitor mechanism and the anti-hypertensive effect produced.

On this subject, the published data available are already so exhaustive as to render further discussion on our part superfluous [10-12].

Worthier of attention are certain details which seem to be typical of the depressant action on PRA brought about by constant oral doses of Labetalol.

Following such a therapeutic procedure, the reduction in PRA can be observed after 5 days' treatment, but the decrease is of little significance, even though the average difference in the reduction is in proportion to the basal levels of the enzyme activiy, whilst the average decrease in plasma aldosterone values is of no statistical importance.

It may be deduced that the renin-angiotensin-aldosterone system is only slightly affected by the oral administration of a daily dose of Labetalol, which is, however, effective in promoting an anti-hypertensive effect.

The action of Labetalol administered at constant daily doses so as to develop an anti-hypertensive response seems to be characterized by a reduced renin-inhibiting activity.

With reference to the renin-inhibiting action

Table V. *Table summarizing the mean deviations of the parameters after 5 days' oral treatment with Labetalol (400 mg/day) in all the patients studied.*

	TOTAL (N=25)		RESPONSIVE (N=13)		NON-RESPONSIVE (N=12)
Supine SBP	18.8±22.2	★★	35±10.2	★★	1.25±17.8
Supine DBP	10±12.6	★★	18.4±7.18	★★	0.8±10.8
Upright SBP	14.2±17.8	★★	28.7±7.23	★★	2.5±17.5
Upright DBP	11±10.5	★★	16.9±5.96	★★	1.26±11.7
HR	3.68±8.24	★★	4.1±6.7	★★	3.5±9.8
Basal PRA	0.2±0.6	★★	0.15±0.68	★★	0.23±0.57
Max. PRA	0.55±1.27	★★	0.51±0.71	★★	0.15±0.73
ALDESTERONE at 8 am	33.7±112.4	★★	41.46±103.7.	★★	25.4±125.3
ALDOSTERONE at 6 pm	57.34±174.9	★★	47.8±169.8	★★	67.58±187.38
Na (P)	— 0.88±3.55	★★	— 1.07±4.5	★★	— 0.75±3.27
K (P)	— 0.116±0.4	★★	— 0.1±0.53	★★	— 0.06±0.24
Na (U)	— 3.96±18.3	★★	— 7.3±23.9	★★	— 0.6±7.15
K (U)	— 0.04±0.53	★★	— 5.3±13.4	★★	— 1.325±3.26

★ $P < 0.05$
★★ $P < 0.01$

of other adrenergic blockers such as Propranolol, which is characterized by a strong inhibiting action on PRA and by an important correlation betwen renin-inhibiting action and anti-hypertensive effect, the inconsistency between the effects of Labetalol on the renin-angiotensin-aldosterone system and its anti-hypertensive effect appears even more striking.

It can thus be affirmed that Labetalol, administered according to our therapeutic procedure, has a moderate renin-inhibiting action which is probably inconsistent with its anti-hypertensive effect.

On the other hand, attention should be drawn to this renin-inhibiting action of Labetalol especially as reflected in its braking action on the PRA increase induced by Furosemide.

To sum up (Table V), oral treatment with 400 mg/day of Labetalol causes a significant reduction in systolic and diastolic BP in both the upright and supine positions, and does not significantly affect heart rate. It has a moderately inhibiting effect on the renin-angiotensin-aldosterone system and also counters the high PRA effect caused by Furosemide.

The anti-hypertensive effect of the drug does not appear to depend on its renin-inhibiting action.

References

1. Boakes A.Y., Knight E.Y., Prichard B.N.C.: Preliminary studies of the pharmacological effects of 5 (-1-hydroxy-2-[(1-methyl 3-phenyl propyl) amino]-ethyl) salicylamide (AH 5158) in man. *Clin. Sci.* 40, 18-20, 1971.
2. Collier J.G., Dawnay N.A.H., Nachev C.H., Robinson B.F.: Clinical investigation of an antagonist at alpha- and beta-adrenoceptors, AH 5158. *Brit. J. Pharmacol.*, 44, 286-293, 1972.
3. Prichard B.N.C. et al. Some hemodynamic effects of the compound AH 5158 compared with propranolol, plus hydralazine, and diazoxide: the use of AH 5158 in the treatment of hypertension. *Clin. Sci. Mol. Med.* 48, Suppl. 2, 97s-100s, 1975.
4. Richards D.A. Pharmacological effects of Labetalol in man. *Brit. J. Clin. Pharmacol.*, 3.4 Suppl. 3, 721-723, 1976.
5. Johnson B.F., Labrooy J., Munroo-Faure A.D.: The antihypertensive efficacy of combined alpha- and beta-adrenoreceptor blockade with phentolamine-oxprenolol or with Labetalol (AH 5158). *Clin. Sci. Mol. Med.* 51, 505-507, 1976.
6. Pugsley D., Armstrong B., Nassim M., Beilin L.J.: Combined alpha- and beta-adrenoreceptor blockade in hypertension: a controlled trial of Labetalol (AH 5158) compared with Propranolol and placebo. *Clin. Sci. Mol. Med.* 4, 15-21, 1976.
7. Bühler F.R., Laragh J.H., Baer L., Vaughan E.D.Jr., Brunner H.R.: Propranolol inhibition of renin secretion. A specific approach to diagnosis and treatment of renin-dependent hypertensive disease. *New Engl. J. Med.* 287, 1209, 1972.
8. Bühler F.R., Laragh J.H., Vaughan E.D.Jr., Brunner H.R., Gavros H., Baer L.: Antihypertensive action of propranolol. Specific antirenin responses in high and normal renin forms of essential, renal, reno-vascular and malignant hypertension. *Am. J. Cardiol.* 32, 511, 1973.
9. Louis W.J., MacNeil J.J., Drummer O., Jarrot B.: Clinical pharmacology of alpha-adrenergic and beta-adrenergic blocking drugs. In: Gross, F. (Ed.): *Modulation of sympathetic tone in the treatment of cardiovascular diseases*. Wien, Hans Huber Publishers, Pag. 25, 1978.
10. Agabiti-Rosei E., Alicandri C., Fariello R., Muiesan G.: Azione antiipertensiva del Labetalolo in rapporto alla attività del sistema adrenergico e del sistema renina-angiotensina. Pp. 117-127. In: Atti Conv. Int. Ipertensione: Nuove prospettive terapeutiche. Venezia, 18-20 Maggio 1978. Glaxo Italia 1978, 269.
11. Salvetti A., Pedrinelli L., Cavasini L., Lera M., Poli L., Sassano P.: L'effetto di dosi crescenti di Labetalolo sul sistema Renina-Angiotensina-Aldosterone e sulla pressione arteriosa di pazienti con ipertensione arteriosa essenziale. Pp. 128-140. In: Atti Conv. Int. Ipertensione: Nuove prospettive terapeutiche. Venezia, 18-20 maggio 1978. Glaxo Italia 1978, 269.
12. Trust P.M. et al.: Effect of blood pressure, angiotensin II and aldosterone concentrations during treatment of severe hypertension with intravenous Labetalol: comparison with propranolol. *Brit. J. Clin. Pharmacol.* 3-4 Suppl. 3, 799-803, 1976.

Hypertension, recent advances and research
edited by M. Condorelli, A. Zanchetti
Cortina International, Verona 1982

The adreno-sympathetic system in essential hypertension

E. AGABITI-ROSEI, C. ALICANDRI, M. BESCHI, E. BONI, M. CASTELLANO, F. FARIELLO, E. MONTINI, M.L.MUIESAN, G. ROMANELLI, G. MUIESAN.
Department V of Clinical Medicine, University of Milan, Civic Hospitals, USLO, Brescia

Key words. Essential Hypertension; Adreno-sympathetic System; Plasma Catecholamines; Haemodynamic Indices; Plasma Renin Activity; Age; Total Peripheral Resistances; Plasma Noradrenalin; Alpha-beta-adrenoceptor Blockade.

Summary. The hypertensive efficacy of drugs blocking the sympathetic system would appear to indicate an increase in adrenergic activity in arterial hypertension. Recent plasma catecholamine assay methods have made it possible to establish a direct correlation between blood pressure and plasma catecholamine levels (PCA). Nevertheless, the way in which sympathetic activity is able to influence the various haemodynamic indices in hypertensive patients has yet to be defined. Our studies have enabled us to note that there exist significant correlations between PCA levels and various haemodynamic indices: PCA levels are directly related to mean blood pressure (MBP) and to Total Peripheral Resistances (TPR) and inversely related to the Systolic Index. A negative, albeit non-significant, relationship has been observed between PCA and Cardiac Output.
The cause-and-effect relationship between the statistically correlated PCA levels and haemodyamic indices appears to be borne out by the fact that basal PCA levels can be used to predict the extent of TPR reduction after alpha-blockade as well as of MBP reduction after combined alpha- and beta-blockade.
In conclusion, the activity of the adrenergic system, as evaluated on the basis of basal PCA concentrations, would appear to be responsible, at least in part, for maintaining elevated pressure values in hypertensive patients, thereby contributing significantly to the degree of peripheral vasoconstriction.

Introduction

The adrenergic nervous system is one of the main factors regulating blood pressure in both normo- and hypertensive patients. At the present time, the most accurate, if not altogether perfect, index for evaluating the activity of the adrenergic system is the assay of the plasma and urinary catecholamines, noradrenalin and adrenalin, which are released by the post-ganglionic adrenergic endings and by the adrenal medulla respectively.

Very high catecholamine values are usually found in pheochromocytoma, a rare form of secondary hypertension in which the high BP values are undoubtedly bound up with the direct cardiovascular effect of noradrenalin and adrenalin. The rôle played by the adrenergic system in essential hypertension is controversial: in this case, circulating catecholamine levels are certainly lower than those found in pheochromocytoma; nonetheless, in pheochromocytoma, the catecholamine - or noradrenalin - plasma levels represent the diluted output of the tumour which is followed only later by the cardiovascular effect, after the passage of amine(s) from the venous to the arterial circulatory system, whereas in essential hypertension, an increase in noradrenalin levels in circulation is a reflection - after considerable dilution - of the release of far smaller quantities of amine which are, however, biologically much more potent because they are discharged directly onto the receptors [27].

The quantification of the catecholamines in the urine provides a reliable assessment of the overall adreno-sympathetic activity for a certain period corresponding to the period of urine collection [28]; moreover, during the urine collection period, physical activity and environmental stresses may vary so that it is difficult to obtain catecholamine values measured in strictly standard conditions in different patients or even in the same patient on different days. Furthermore, since catecholamines are eliminated largely by glomerular filtration [22], the determination of noradrenalin and adrenalin levels in the urine can supply reliable data corresponding to the real activity of the adrenergic system, only in patients with absolutely normal renal function [27].

The introduction of sensitive and repetitive methods for assaying noradrenalin and adrenalin, even in small volumes of plasma [7, 20, 25] has made possibile a sufficiently accurate evaluation of the adrenergic system.

In fact, it has been shown that noradrenalin and adrenalin in the plasma increase in proportion, in all pathophysiological conditions which are accompanied by a more or less intense adrenergic stimulation, such as the standing position, dynamic or isometric physical exercise, Valsalva's manoeuvre, the cold pressor test, etc. Moreover, when plasma catecholamines were determined on different days in the same patient examined in standard conditions, the results obtained proved to overlap [6].

On this basis, those hypertensive patients who have high BP levels attributable, at least in part, to the adrenergic system, will most likely have above-normal levels of catecholamines in circulation. On the other hand, apart from the possible differences between normotensives and hypertensives with regard to the plasma concentration of catecholamines, it is extremely important to establish whether or not there is a causal relationship between adrenergic activity and haemodynamic characteristics in patients with essential hypertension; extremely important to establish whether or not there is a causal relationship between adrenergic activiy and haemodynamic characteristics in patients with essential hypertension; in other words, it is important to find out whether catecholamines have a direct bearing on BP values and if, by eliminating the biological effect of noradrenalin and/or adrenalin in circulation by the use of drugs, BP values can be reduced in proportion to the level of activity of the adrenergic system.

These aspects of the study concerning the relationship between adrenergic activity and essential hypertension will be examined below on the basis of the results of personal studies and in relation to data available in literature.

Plasma concentrations of catecholamines in essential hypertensives and in normotensive subjects

The assay of the noradrenalin and adrenalin concentrations in patients with varying levels of essential hypertension in comparison with those of normotensive subjects has been the topic of more than 30 publications [14]; about 90% of these studies showed higher plasma concentrations of noradrenalin in hypertensives than in normotensives, but the difference was statistically significant in only about half of them.

Similarly, our group verified, some years ago, significantly higher plasma concentrations of adrenalin and, especially, of noradrenalin in hypertensive subjects than in normotensive subjects of the same age, both in the supine and upright positions [27] (Fig. 1).

There are various possible explanations of the relative discrepancies in the results obtained in these different studies. A rigorous uniformity in the experimental conditions in which the blood samples are taken is of vital importance for the accurate calculation of catecholamines: the sodium content in the diet [24], the length of time spent in the supine or upright position before the sample was taken, the types of drugs used previously and the

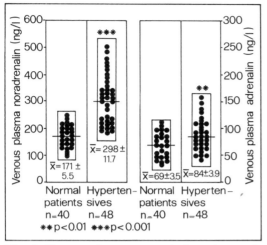

Fig. 1. Venous plasma concentrations (mean ± s.e.m.) of noradrenalin and adrenalin in 48 patients whit stable essential hypertension and in 40 normal subjects.[27]

time of their withdrawal, the patients' smoking and drinking habits, possible associated symptoms or life-style of the normotensive subjects, the time elapsing between the blood-sampling and the catecholamine assay are all factors which may have a considerable influence on the results and which are not always carefully checked in such studies[5]. Consideration should also be given to the age of the subjects; Lake et al.[18], in fact, pointed out that noradrenalin increases with age and maintained that the high values found in hypertensives in previous studies were due to the fact that the control group of normotensives were all younger; in actual fact, later studies were able to confirm the significant positive correlation between noradrenalin and age whilst other scholars have observed that noradrenalin increases with age in normotensive subjects but not in hypertensives[3].

After analyzing the data published in 32 studies, on a population of 1496 hypertensives and 1085 normotensives, Goldstein[14] was able to draw the conclusion that plasma noradrenalin values are, on the whole, significantly higher in patients with essential hypertension (P 0.05) in comparison with normotensive subjects. Taken all together, the results of the different studies certainly suggest - even if they

do not prove - that, on the basis of plasma noradrenalin values, a group of hypertensive patients has increased adrenergic activity in comparison with the normotensive subjects.

Most of the researchers noticed significant differences between hypertensive and normotensive subjects, especially with regard to noradrenalin, to which they consequently dedicated their attention, rather than to adrenalin. Only a few of the studies, concerning a more limited number of patients, reported a high concentration of plasma adrenalin[13]: however, the differences between hypertensives and normotensives were quite small and have not been confirmed by more recent studies.

Certainly, at the present time, the available assay methods appear to be more sensitive and reproducible as far as noradrenalin is concerned; but the possibility cannot be excluded that in the future there will be more precise assay methods permitting a better assessment of the rôle of adrenalin, as an index of adrenergic activity, in essential hypertension.

Interrelationships between catecholamines, BP and age in essential hypertension

The presence of above-normal plasma noradrenalin values in hypertensive patients does not necessarily imply that the adrenergic system can influence BP values, thereby determining, at least in part, the gravity of the hypertensive condition.

We have studied the possible interrelationships between plasma catecholamines and BP, also in relation to age, in a group of 94 essential hypertension patients (44 females and 50 males) aged between 24 and 66 years. According to the WHO classification, 52 patients belonged to class I and 39 to class II; the remaining 3 were considered class III because they had retinous exudates at the fundus oculi. All had normal renal function. No patient exhibited any clinical signs of left venticular insufficiency. Their hypertension was defined as essential on the basis of the usual clinical, laboratory and instrument tests.

Other therapies had been withdrawn at least 4 weeks earlier and the patients had been on a

15

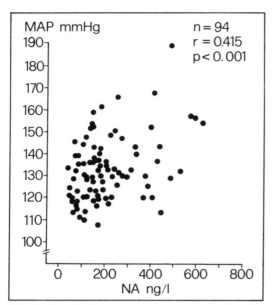

Fig. 2. Correlation between plasma noradrenalin (NA) and mean blood pressure (MAP) in 94 essential hypertension patients.

normal sodium (⌐ 120 mEq/24 hrs) and potassium (⌐ 80 mEq/24 hrs) diet for 3-5 days. The examinations were always carried out in the morning, before the patients had eaten and after they had been lying down for at least an hour. The plasma catecholamines were assessed by means of the sensitive and repeatable fluorimetric method of Renzini et al. [25]. The results obtained with this method virtually overlap those obtained using isotopic methods [20], and the values presented in most cases represent the average of the two readings.

In this large group of hypertensive patients a positive correlation (r = 0.41) of statistical significance (p < 0.001) was found between plasma noradrenalin and mean BP (obtained by adding 1/3 of the pressure differential to the diastolic BP) (Fig. 2).

Similar correlation coefficients were also observed considering systolic or diastolic BP on the one hand and plasma noradrenalin on the other. No significant correlation was found, however, between BP values and adrenalin. A positive correlation between plasma noradrenalin and BP with coefficients resembling ours has been observed by other authors

[3, 4, 9, 17, 21, 29] in groups of various size and nature. Generally speaking, given that the adrenergic system is not the only factor regulating BP, extremely high correlation coefficients cannot be expected, but all these observations seem to suggest quite clearly that increased adrenergic activity in hypertensive patients not suffering from renal or cardiac impairment is associated with higher BP values.

In the patients participating in our study a positive correlation was observed between age and systolic BP (r = 0.40), but not between age and diastolic BP (r = 0.08); moreover, no significant correlation was found between age and plasma noradrenalin. The influence of the adrenergic system on BP thus appears to be independent of age.

Interrelationships between catecholamines and renin in essential hypertension

It is well known that the adrenergic system is one of the factors capable of regulating the release of renin [15, 29]. Moreover, it has been suggested that an increased adrenal-sympathetic activity may be involved in the pathogenesis of essential hypertension with high renin levels [9], whereas reduced adrenergic activity was observed in some patients with low renin levels [10]. In 89 essential hypertension patients aged between 24 and 66 years, studied under the above-described standard conditions, we simultaneously determined the plasma concentrations of catecholamines and the plasma renin activity (PRA) using the radioimmunoassay method of Haber and colleagues [16] in modified form. A positive correlation (r = 0.34) of statistical significance (p < 0.01) was observed between PRA and plasma noradrenalin measured in the supine position (Fig. 3).

The correlation coefficient is not high, which means that, in basal conditions, the adrenergic system may indeed have some influence on the release of renin but this influence is not decisive. No correlation was noted between adrenalin and PRA.

Since with the sodium content of the diet used in this study normal PRA values range between 0.5 and 3 ng/ml/h, the patients were divided into 3 groups according to their renin

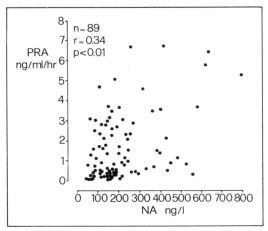

Fig. 3. Correlation between plasma noradrenalin (NA) and plasma renin activity (PRA) in 89 essential hypertension patients.

levels - low, normal, or high. Above-normal plasma noradrenalin values were observed in 40% of the cases (6/15) with low renin levels (Fig. 4). On average, however, the noradrenalin values were significantly higher only in patients with high renin levels, whereas no difference was observed between groups of patients with low or normal renin levels. Furthermore, the patients studied who had low renin levels also had a significantly lower heart rate, and were much older. Altogether, these data suggest that patients with low renin levels may

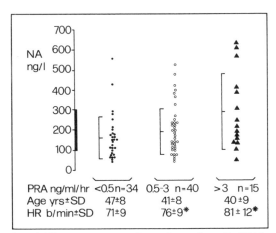

PRA ng/ml/hr	<0.5 n=34	0.5-3 n=40	>3 n=15
Age yrs±SD	47±8	41±8	40±9
HR b/min±SD	71±9	76±9*	81±12*

Fig. 4. Plasma concentrations of noradrenalin (NA) in 3 groups of patients subdivided on the basis of their PRA: low, normal, or high.

have not so much a lower adrenergic activity as a lower beta-receptor sensitivity, both renal and cardiac, to the same adrenergic stimulation. This reduced sensitivity, as suggested by Bertel et al. [3], may be in relation to the more advanced age.

On the other hand, a considerable percentage of the patients with high renin levels seems to have increased adrenergic activity, as indicated by the circulating levels of noradrenalin. In any case, renin levels and, consequently angiotensin II levels, may contribute in part to the high BP values found in patients with high renin levels and high plasma concentrations of noradrenalin.

Plasma catecholamines and haemodynamic characteristics in patients with essential hypertension

In our study, plasma noradrenalin proved to be directly related to BP in hypertensive patients. The entity of the BP values is determined basically by the relationship between circulatory output and peripheral resistances. Since the adrenergic system is capable of both increasing cardiac output and inducing vasoconstriction, we carried out a haemodynamic study on 41 of the above patients (25 males and 16 females) aged between 30 and 66 years, with the aim of examining the possible correlations between plasma catecholamines and the various haemodynamic indices. In 27 patients cardiac output was determined using the dye-dilution method (indocyanine green) and the curves were calculated according to the Stewart-Hamilton technique. In 14 patients cardiac output was determined using the thermodilution method. The values obtained by the two methods overlap (personal data not published).

The total peripheral vascular resistances were calculated on the basis of the cardiac index and expressed in units (V/cm^2). The details of the methods used are described elsewhere [1,2]. Also in this subgroup of patients a positive statistically significant correlation was observed between noradrenalin and mean BP (Fig. 5).

No correlation was noted between plasma

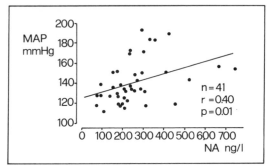

Fig. 5. Correlation between plasma noradrenalin (NA) and mean blood pressure in 41 essential hypertension patients subjected to haemodynamic examinations.

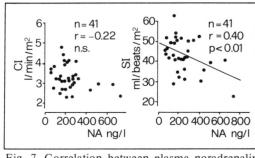

Fig. 7. Correlation between plasma noradrenalin (NA) and (left) cardiac index (CI), and between NA and stroke index (SI) in 41 essential hypertension patients subjected to haemodynamic examinations.

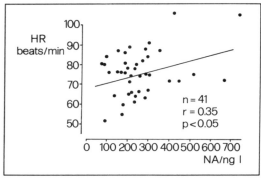

Fig. 6. Correlation between plasma noradrenalin (NA) and heart rate (HR) in 41 essential hypertension patients subjected to haemodynamic examinations.

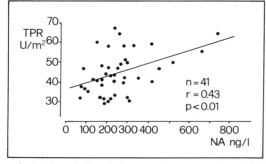

Fig. 8. Correlation between plasma noradrenalin (NA) and total peripheral resistances (TPR) in 41 essential hypertension patients subjected to haemodynamic examinations.

noradrenalin and cardiac index (Fig. 7); this seems to be the consequence of the fact that plasma noradrenalin is directly related to heart rate (Fig. 6) and inversely related to the systolic index (Fig. 7). A positive and statistically significant correlation, conversely, was found between plasma noradrenalin and total peripheral resistences (Fig. 8). There did not appear to be any correlation between adrenalin and the various haemodynamic indices. Moreover, in the group of stable hypertension patients we studied, the influence of the adrenergic system on BP seems to operate basically through the regulation of the degree of peripheral vasoconstriction.

These results give a vaster significance to some of our preceding observations and con-

form with the findings of Mime et al. [21]. These authors also showed that in some younger borderline hypertensives, a high adrenergic tone may be accompanied by greater cardiac output; similarly, in younger patients wih borderline hypertension, high renin and catecholamine levels, Esler et al. [11, 12] found a significantly greater cardiac output than in patients with normal renin and plasma catecholamine levels.

These findings do not contradict our results as they may be interpreted on the basis of those presented by Bertel et al. [3], according to whom, as mentioned above, increased BP values and increased age in patients with essential hypertension seem to be associated with a steady reduction in the sensitivity and/or responsiveness of the beta-adrenergic receptors, with consequent greater peripheral vasoconstriction mediated by the alpha-adrenergic receptors. Therefore, in younger patients, with less serious hypertension, adrenergic activity may influence both the amount of the circulation flow and the peripheral resistences, whereas in older patients, with fixed hypertension, the main haemodynamic effect of increased adrenergic activity consists in greater peripheral vasoconstriction.

Effect of drug blocking of alpha- and beta-adrenoceptors

The correlations observed between noradrenalin and the different haemodynamic indices, even if statistically significant, do not necessarily imply a cause-effect relationship. One useful way of seeking confirmation or otherwise of such a relationship is to study the haemodynamic effects induced by drugs which selectively block the adrenergic nervous system, also in relation to the basal values of circulating catecholamines and/or their modifications following treatment. A few years ago, Louis et al. [19] demonstrated that the patients who had the highest BP values gave the greatest hypotensive response and, at the same time, also the most consistent reduction in plasma concentrations of noradrenalin after the administration of the ganglionic blocker, Pentolinium. Likewise, Esler et al. [11] observed in borderline hypertension subjects, that the drug blocking of the autonomic nervous system, obtained by the successive administration of Propranolol, Atropine and Phentolamine, brought about greater reductions in BP and in the peripheral resistances in those subjects whose basal plasma noradrenalin and PRA were higher.

We used Labetalol, a drug known for its simultaneous alpha-and beta-blocking action on adrenoceptors, in 27 of the above-described patients (12 males and 15 females) aged between 30 and 60. In 18 of them, haemodynamic examinations were carried out before treatment and 30 min. after administration of the drug. Administered intravenously at a dose of 100 mg, Labetalol effectively blocks both

the alpha- and beta-adrenoceptors, as demonstrated by the fact that, with Valsalva's manoeuvre, both the dip frequency increase and the BP increase to overshoot are virtually inhibited by the administration of the drug [23].

In the whole group of 27 hypertensives studied, the administration of Labetalol, on average, produced a considerable and significant reduction in systolic and diastolic BP, which was apparent only 5 min. later and which lasted, virtually unaltered, for more than an hour [2]. In this group of 27 patients, the systolic, diastolic and mean BP reductions, whether considered as absolute or percentage values, proved to be closely connected to the basal plasma noradrenalin values (Fig. 9).

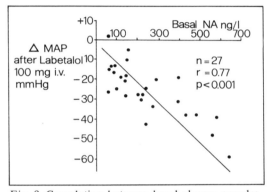

Fig. 9. Correlation between basal plasma noradrenalin (NA) and the mean arterial pressure (MAP) reduction after an intravenous dose of 100 mg of Labetalol in 27 essential hypertension patients.

Even heart rate decreased in a statistically significant way after treatment with Labetalol. Moreover, in some patients, namely those with higher basal noradrenalin levels, heart rate underwent a greater reduction; thus it was possible to note a significant correlation between basal concentration of plasma noradrenalin and the proportions of the decrease in HR after the administration of Labetalol (r = 0.48, p < 0.02) (Fig. 10).

From the haemodynamic point of view, the intravenous administration of Labetalol causes a reduction in BP values mainly due to a peripheral vasodilation mechanism. In fact, in the 18 patients subjected to the haemodynamic

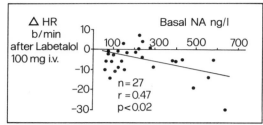

Fig. 10. Correlation between basal plasma noradrenalin (NA) and the reduction in heart rate (HR) after an intravenous dose of 100 mg of Labetalol in 27 essential hypertension patients.

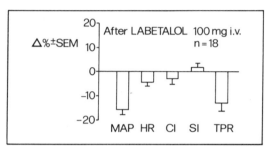

Fig. 11. Percentage modifications of the various haemodynamic indices (mean ± s.e.m.) after 100 mg of Labetalol i.v. in 18 essential hypertension patients. MAP = mean arterial pressure; HR = heart rate; CI = cardiac index; SI = systolic index; TPR = total peripheral resistances.

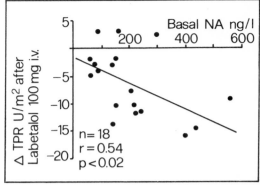

Fig. 12. Correlation between basal plasma noradrenalin (NA) and the reduction in the total peripheral resistances (TPR) estimated after the i.v. administration of 100 mg of Labetalol in 18 essential hypertension patients.

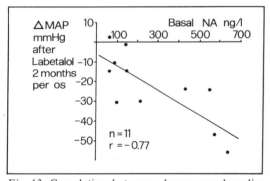

Fig. 13. Correlation between plasma noradrenalin (NA) and the reduction in mean arterial pressure (MAP) after Labetalol per os for 1-2 months in 11 essential hypertension patients.

study, the circulatory output did not, on average, show any significant alteration, whereas the reduction in BP values was demonstrated to be correlated to the reduction in the estimated total peripheral resistances (Fig. 11). Furthermore, the amount of the reduction in these peripheral resistances proved greater the higher the basal values of plasma noradrenalin (Fig. 12).

Eleven patients were given oral treatment with Labetalol for a period of 1-2 months, at a maximum dose of 1,200 mg/day and in any case enough to reduce BP values, if possible, without causing side effects. In these patients, too, the reduction in the BP values, after chronic treatment, was greater in those patients who had higher basal levels of plasma noradrenalin ($r = 0.77$, p   0.01) (Fig. 13). The blocking effects of the drug on the alpha-

and beta-adrenoceptors thus provides confirmation of the participation of the adrenergic system, in varying degrees according to the case, in controlling the various haemodynamic parameters in hypertensive patients, especially by determining the degree of peripheral vasoconstriction.

Conclusions

Many studies have demonstrated that the activity of the adrenergic system, as estimated on the basis of the plasma concentrations of noradrenalin and adrenalin, is significantly greater in patients suffering from essential hypertension.

Since catecholamines are present in the plasma in small quantities and since they reflect only partially the active quantity at the receptor sites, in order to observe significant differences between normotensives and hypertensives and define the possible rôle of the adrenergic system in determining the haemodynamic characteristics of hypertensive patients, the methods used must be sensitive and repeatable, and the experimental conditions of the various studies must be strictly uniform. Failure to abide by these rules may well be the main reason for the discrepancies in the results of the different studies, especially with regard to the existence of a significant difference in plasma catecholamine concentrations as between normo- and hypertensive subjects.

On the other hand, since hypertension is fundamentally a haemodynamic alteration whereby every circulatory output value brings an undesired increase in the peripheral resistances, it is vital to know if, and to what degree, the adrenergic system affects the haemodynamic characteristics of different hypertensive patients.

In our study group of patients with stable hypertension we noted that plasma noradrenalin, rather than adrenalin, is correlated in a significant way to the various haemodynamic indices of the hypertensive patients. Our results show that the adrenergic system may, at least in part, directly affect BP values, determining above all the degree of peripheral vasoconstriction in a group of patients with stable essential hypertension. In fact, plasma noradrenalin proved to have a direct and statistically significant connection with BP, heart rate and peripheral resistances and to be inversely related to the systolic index. Other studies have shown that in younger patients cardiac output as well as peripheral resistances may be higher when plasma noradrenalin is higher. The recognition of the presence of excess adrenergic activity in stabilized hypertensive patients does not explain whether it is a cause or a consequence of the hypertensive state, and this might be the topic of future studies.

Certainly, the adrenergic system is not the only factor responsible for maintaining high BP values, perhaps not even in patients with higher plasma levels of noradrenalin; for example, in patients with excess adrenergic activity an increase in PRA has not infrequently been observed, and it is possible that in these cases the activation of the renin-angiotensin system may contribute to the degree of hypertension. Moreover, the importance of the alterations of the arterial walls, of sodium, and of the quantity and distribution of the volume of extracellular liquids is well known and must not be underestimated.

More precise information about the rôle of the adrenergic system in arterial hypertension can be obtained by devising sufficiently accurate methods for assessing the number and sensitivity of the adrenoceptors, and by a better definition of the processes of release and metabolism of the neutrotransmitter at vascular area level, which are particularly important for regulating BP values.

Even now, however, the measurement of plasma catecholamine levels in hypertensive patients is not meaningless. We have seen that the higher the plasma concentration of noradrenaline, the greater the reduction in BP and in peripheral vasodilation, after simultaneous blocking of the alpha- and beta-adrenoceptors. This proves that the correlations observed are significant not only statistically but probably also from a biological point of view.

In practice, the measurement of plasma noradrenalin may make it possible to foresee the extent of the BP decrease after alpha- and beta-blocking treatment. Alternatively, the degree of BP reduction after the administration of an alpha- and beta-blocking drug can indicate the level of activity of the adrenergic system and therefore provide useful pointers for the most suitable therapy in each individual case.

References

1. Agabiti-Rosei E., Alicandri C., Fariello R., Muiesan G.: Catecholamines and haemodynamics in fixed es-

sential hypertension. *Clin. Sci. Mol. Med.*, 57, 1935 1979.

2. Agabiti-Rosei E., Alicandri C., Beschi M., Castellano M., Fariello R., Montini E., Muiesan M.L., Romanelli G., Muiesan G.: Plasma catecholamines and the hypotensive effect of Labetalol. *Brit. J. Clin. Pharmacol.* (in press).

3. Bertel D., Bühler F.R., Kiowski W., Lütold B.E.: Decreased beta-adrenoreceptor responsiveness as related to age, blood pressure and plasma catecholamines in patients with essential hypertension. *Hypertension*, 2, 130, 1980.

4. Brecht H.M., Schoeppe W.: Relation of plasma noradrenaline to blood pressure, age, sex and sodium balance in patients with stable essential hypertension and in normotensive subjects. *Clin. Sci. Mol. Med*, 55, 81s, 1978.

5. Carruthers M., Taggart P., Conway N., Bates D.: Validity of plasma catecholamine estimations. *Lancet*, 2, 62, 1970.

6. Cousineau D., Lapointe L., De Champlain G.: Circulating catecholamines and systolic time intervals in normotensive and hypertensive patients with and without left ventricular hypertrophy. *Am. Heart J.*, 96, 227, 1978.

7. Da Prada M., Zürcher G.: Simultaneous radioenzymatic determination of plasma and tissue adrenaline, noradrenaline and dopamine within the femtomole range. *Life Sci.*, 18, 1161-1174, 1976.

8. De Champlain J., Cousineau D.: Lack of correlation between age and circulating catecholamines in hypertensive subjects. *New Engl. J. Med.*, 297, 12, 672 1977.

9. De Quattro V., Miura Y., Meijer D.: Increased plasma catecholamines in high-renin hypertension. *Am. J. Cardiol.*, 38, 801 1976.

10. Esler M., Zweifler A. Randall O., Julius S., Bennett J., Rydelek P., Cohen E., De Quattro V.: Suppression of sympathetic nervous function in low-renin essential hypertension. *Lancet*. 2, 115, 1976.

11. Esler M., Julius S., Randall O., De Quattro V., Zweifler A.: High-renin essential hypertension: adrenergic cardiovascular correlates. *Clin. Sci. Mol. Med.*, 51, 181s, 1976.

12. Esler M., Juliis S., Zweifler A., Randall O., Harburg E., Gardiner H., De Quattro V.: Mild high-renin essential hypertension: a neurogenic human hypertension? *New Eng. J. Med.*, 296, 405, 1977.

13. Franco-Morselli R., Elghozi J. L., Joly E., Di Giulio S., Meyer P.: Increased plasma adrenaline concentrations in benign essential hypertension. *Brit. Med. J.*, 2, 1251, 1977.

14. Goldstein D.S.: Plasma norepinephrine in essential hypertension - A study of the studies. *Hypertension*, 3, 48, 1981.

15. Gordon R.D., Kuchel O., Liddle G.W. Island D.P.: Rôle of the sympathetic nervous system in regulating renin and aldosterone production in man. *J. Clin. Invest.*, 46, 599, 1967.

16. Haber E., Koerner T., Page L.B., Kliman B., Purnode A.: Application of a radioimmunoassay for angiotensin I to the physiologic measurements of plasma renin activity in normal human subjects. *J. Clin. Endocr.*, 29, 1349, 1969.

17. Hong Tai Eng F.W., Huber-Smith M., McCann D.S.: The rôle of sympathetic activity in normal-renin essential hypertension. *Hypertension*, 2, 14, 1980.

18. Lake C.R., Ziegler M.G., Coleman M.D., Kopin J.K.: Age-adjusted plasma norepinephrine levels are similar in normotensive and hypertensive subjects. *New Engl. J. Med.*, 296, 208, 1977.

19. Louis W.J., Doyle A.E., Anavekar S.: Plasma norepinephrine levels in essential hypertension. *New Engl. J. Med.*, 288, 599, 1973.

20. Miura Y., Campese V., De Quattro V., Meijer B.: Plasma catecholamines via an improved fluorimetric assay: comparison with an enzyme method. *J. Lab. Clin. Med.*, 89, 421, 1977.

21. Miura Y., Kobayashi K., Sakuma H., Tomioka H., Adachi M., Yoshinaga K.: Plasma noradrenaline concentrations and haemodynamics in the early stage of essential hypertension. *Clin. Sci. Mol. Med.*, 55, 69s, 1978.

22. Muiesan G., Valori C., Brunori C., Corea L., Gigli G.: Studies of renal clearance of adrenaline and noradrenaline in man. *IVth International Congress of Nephrology*, Stockholm, p. 399, 1969.

23. Muiesan G., Agabiti-Rosei E., Alicandri C., Fariello R.: Sistema nervoso adrenergico ed ipertensione; In: *Ipertensione arteriosa in nefrologia*. p. 19. Milano, Masson, 1981.

24. Nicholls M.G., Kiowski W., Zweifler A.J., Julius S., Schork M.A., Greenhouse J.: Plasma norepinephrine variations with dietary sodium intake. *Hypertension*, 2, 29, 1980.

25. Renzini V., Brunori C.A., Valori C.: A sensitive and specific fluorimetric method for the determination of noradrenaline and adrenaline in human plasma. *Clin. Chim. Acta*, 30, 587, 1970.

26. Robertson D., Johnson G.A., Robertson R.M., Nies A.S., Shand D.G., Oates J.A.: Comparative assessment of stimuli that release neuronal and adrenomedullary catecholamines in man. *Circulation*, 59, 637, 1979.

27. Valori C., Pinchi G. Brancifiori M., Agabiti-Rosei E.: Ruolo del sistema simpatico adrenergico e riflessi diagnostici e terapeutici. *Atti Simposio su Ipertensione arteriosa. 37° Congr. Soc. Ital. Cardiol.*, p. 29, 1976.

28. Von Euler U.S.: A specific sympathomimetic ergone in adrenergic nerve fibres (sympathin): relations to adrenaline and noradrenaline. *Acta Physiol. Scand.*, 12, 73, 1946.

29. Winer N., Chokshi D.S., Walkenhorst W.G.: Effects of cyclic AMP, sympathomimetic amines, and adrenergic receptor antagonists on renin secretion. *Circ. Res.*, 29, 239, 1971.

Hypertension, recent advances and research
edited by M. Condorelli, A. Zanchetti
Cortina International, Verona 1982

The influence of the administration of Labetalol on the endocrinal activity of the pancreas in diabetic and non-diabetic hypertensives

G.D. BOMPIANI, G.A. CERASOLA, M.L. MORICI, M. DONATELLI

3rd Institute of General Clinical and Therapeutic Medicine, University of Palermo

Key words. Labetalol; Endocrinal Activity; Pancreas; Diabetic Hypertensives; Non-diabetic Hypertensives; Alpha-beta-adrenoceptors; Glucose Metabolism; Oral Glucose Tolerance Test; Serum Insulin; Glucagon; Plasma Renin Activity; NEFA; Plasma Catecholamines; Urinary Catecholamines.

Summary The knowledge that the mechanisms regulating the endocrinal activity of the pancreas are mediated by alpha- and beta-adrenoceptors with divergent action led the authors to study the effects of Labetalol, a non-selective alpha- and beta-blocking drug, on the glucose metabolism.

The subjects studied were 16 hypertensives, 10 of whom had glucose metabolism disorders and 6 with no metabolic illness.

The study was carried out by means of the execution of the oral glucose tolerance test (O.G.T.T.) with the determination of serum insulin, glucose and glucagon before treatment and on the 10th day of administration of Labetalol at the dose of 300 mg/day.

Blood pressure, heart rate, plasma renin activity, NEFA and the urinary and plasma catecholamines were also assessed before and during treatment.

The administration of the drug brought about a significant reduction in systolic and diastolic blood pressure in all patients examined and a non-significant decrease in heart rate and PRA.

The glucose, insulin and glucagon curves of the 6 control hypertensives (non-diabetic) did not undergo any significant change as a result of treatment with Labetalol. The values of the glucose curves of patients with overt diabetes seem to decrease, but generally not in a significant manner, after treatment, whilst the insulin and glucagon curves of the same patients remain more or less unchanged. The insulin curves of those patients with impaired glucose tolerance decrease significantly at the 90th and 120th minutes and this decrease is accompanied by a non-significant lowering of the glucose values.

The NEFA are reduced moderately in all subjects, both diabetic and non-diabetic, after treatment with the drug.

The daily excretion of urinary catecholamines, determined by the fluorometric method, seems to increase after Labetalol; this increase is not confirmed, however, by the radioenzymic assay of the plasma catecholamines which, on the contrary, show a slight decrease.

The authors discuss the results obtained.

Introduction

In recent years, many studies have been carried out, on both animals and man, to find out whether the beta-adrenoreceptor blocking drugs have metabolic effects, besides their well-known cardio-vascular action.

Studies made a few years ago by Porte [21-22], Cerasi [3], Robertson [24] and other authors have proved that there is a receptor system at endocrine pancreas level which, when stimulated by isoproterenol or other beta-mimetic substances, causes a noticeable increase in insulin secretion, and that the pancreatic receptor for glucose is a beta-receptor.

Subsequent observations and clinical experiments, however, have shown that endocrine acitivity regulation depends not only on the rôle of the beta-receptors but also on the less important rôle of the alpha-adrenoreceptors. In fact, stimulation of the pancreatic alpha-receptors by means of adrenalin or noradrenalin infusion or during pheochromocytoma, inhibits the insulin response to glucose and, conversely, the infusion of phentolamine or other alpha-blockers causes an increase in both basal insulinemia and the insulin response to glucose or to arginine [4-5-20-22-25-40].

Consequently, the effects of the adrenergic stimulation and blockade on insulin secretion are the following:
1) the alpha-receptor blockade increases production
2) the stimulation of the alpha-receptors suppresses production
3) the beta-receptor blockade suppresses production
4) the stimulation of the beta-receptors increases production.

Finally, the most recent research, either administering selective and non-selective beta-stimulating substances or using selective and non-selective beta-blocking drugs for the beta$_1$-receptors, has enabled many authors to assert that the insulin response to glucose is not mediated by beta$_1$-adrenoreceptors but most probably by beta$_2$-adrenoreceptors. [6-7-13-15-17-29]

These physiopathological premises plus the wide-scale current use of beta-adrenoreceptor blockers in the long-term treatment of ischaemic heart diseases and arterial hypertension, pathologies increasingly associated with glucose metabolism alterations, have encouraged the search for the adverse effects on metabolism possibly brought about by the chronic administration of a simultaneously alpha- and beta-blocking substance on the adrenergic receptors, which is non-selective and has no intrinsic sympatheticomimetic activity.

Methods

The group studied consisted of 10 patients aged between 25 and 55 years, with essential hypertension and overt non-insulin-dependent diabetes, or impaired glucose tolerance, and 6 hypertensive control patients, of the same age group and sex, with no form of metabolic alteration.

All patients were hospitalized and kept, for the entire duration of the trial, on a standard diet containing 120 mEq of sodium, 90 mEq of potassium and 185 grams/day of carbohydrates.

During the first 10 days of hospitalization, the patients were given only a placebo in three oral administrations daily, and were checked at least twice a day for their heart rate and blood pressure.

At the end of the wash-out period, samples were taken for routine blood tests and for the study of kidney and liver function, and the cardiological examination was carried out.

The following morning, after 12 hours' fasting, a needle cannula was inserted in the patient's antecubital vein, and after an hour of total rest samples were taken to determine the serum concentrations of electrolytes, catecholamines, glucose, insulin, glucagon and basal NEFA. Immediately afterwards, the patients were given an oral administration of 100 grams of glucose dissolved in 150 ml of water and samples were taken for assessing serum glucose, insulin and glucagon at minutes 30, 60, 90, 120, 150 and 180.

The same day, urine collection was begun for the determination of the electrolytes and of the urinary catecholamines, and the following morning a sample was taken, after orthostatic stimulation, for determing the PRA.

The patients were then started on oral treatment with Labetalol at the rate of 300 mg/day per os in 3 administrations for a period of 10 days.

Clinical checks were carried out every day and on the 9th and 10th days of treatment samples were collected for determining serum and urinary electrolytes, plasma and urinary catecholamines, serum NEFA, PRA, serum glucose, insulin and glucagon before and after

Table I. *Summary of the trial programme.*

HYPERTENSIVE PATIENTS n = 16 AGE 25 - 55 yrs.)
WITHOUT DIABETES n = 6 WITH IMPAIRED GLUCOSE TOLERANCE (IGT) n = 5 WITH OVERT DIABETES n = 5
days   —10   0   10
WASH-OUT   LABETALOL mg 300 die

SERUM ELECTROLYTES
P.R.A.
NEFA
URINARY CATECHOLAMINES
PLASMA CATECHOLAMINES
O.G.T.T.: BLOOD GLUCOSE
             INSULIN
             GLUCAGON

SERUM ELECTROLYTES
P.R.A.
NEFA
URINARY CATECHOLAMINES
PLASMA CATECHOLAMINES
O.G.T.T.: BLOOD GLUCOSE
             INSULIN
             GLUCAGON

glucose loading, using the same methods as for the baseline check (Table I).

Serum glucose was assessed by means of the (glucose-oxydase) enzymic method.

The NEFA were determined using the Carlo Erba colorimetric method.

Serum insulin was calculated by radioimmunoassay on resin, using the Dow-Lepetit kit.

Serum glucagon was determined by the double-antibody method, using the Bio-Data kit.

PRA was assayed by generating angiotensin I in ng/ml/h, using the Dow-Lepetit kit.

The fluorometric method was used for the determination of the urinary catecholamines.

The plasma catecholamines were determined with the radioenzymic method (H₃ CO-MT), by means of thin-layer chromatography using the Upjohn kit.

Blood presure was measured twice daily, on the right arm, after at least 10 minutes in the supine position, using a mercury manometer with a cuff 26 cm long by 12.5 cm wide; diastolic BP was identified with Korotkoff phase 5.

Heart rate was studied at the centrum cordis in the supine position, immediately after each blood pressure reading. In calculating the results, the mean values recorded during the wash-out period and during the treatment period were considered separately for these two parameters.

Student's "t" was used to assess the statistical significance of the results.

Results

The results of our study show first of all that the administration of the drug, at the given doses, brought about a steady and significant reduction in both systolic and diastolic BP in all patients examined. The mean reduction in systolic BP was from 163.4 ± 6.4 SD to $148.1 \pm$ SD (P   0.001), whilst for diastolic BP it was from 99 ± 6.9 SD to 92.1 ± 6.2 SD (P   0.01) (Fig. 1).

Mean heart rate was reduced in all patients examined from 76.9 ± 11.1 SD to 71.3 ± 9.8

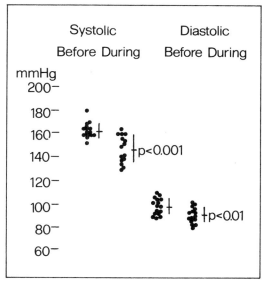

Fig. 1. Behaviour of mean systolic and diastolic blood pressure of each patient, before and during treatment with Labetalol (Mean±SD n = 16).

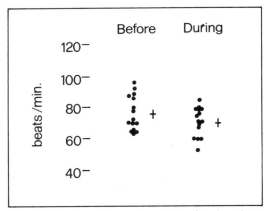

Fig. 2. Behaviour of mean heart rate of each patient, before and during treatment with Labetalol (Mean ±SD n = 16).

SD after treatment, but this decrease was not significant (Fig. 2).

PRA, after orthostatic stimulation, reveals a mean decrease from 0.86 to 0.49 ng/ml/h; though considerable, this decrease is not statistically significant (Fig. 3).

With regard to the metabolic study of our non-diabetic hypertensive patients, the basal glucose values and the trend of the glucose curve, both before and during treatment, more or less overlap. The behaviour of serum insu-

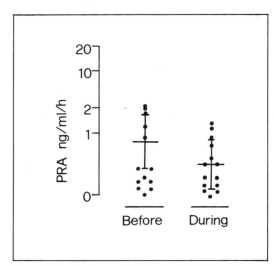

Fig. 3. Evaluation of PRA in diabetic and non-diabetic hypertensives, before treatment and on the 10th day of treatment with Labetalol (Mean ± S.E.M. n = 16).

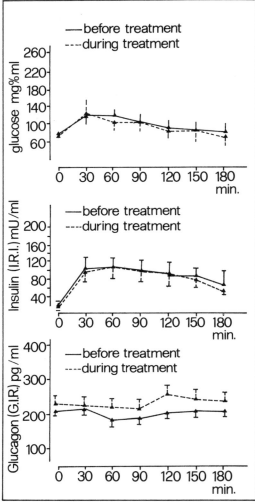

Fig. 4. Behaviour of glucose, insulin and glucagon, before and after treatment with Labetalol (Mean ± S.E.M. n =16).

lin and glucagon in the same patients is similar: the insulin and glucagon curves in fact show no significant point of difference in relation to the treatment (Fig. 4).

With reference to the 10 hypertensive patients with impaired carbohydrate metabolism, the glucose curve plotted during treatment reveals a reduction, though not significant, in the glucose values along the entire curve profile. No difference is observed, in relation to the treatment, in the insulin and glucagon curves (Fig. 5).

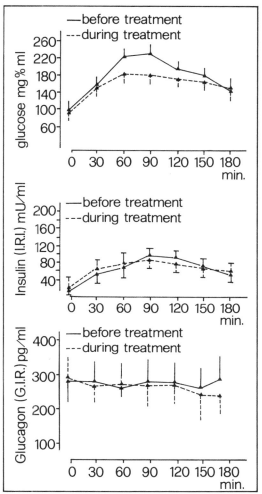

Fig. 5. Serum glucose insulin and glucagon throughout the O.G.T.T. curve in hypertensives with metabolic disorders, before treatment and on the 10th day of treatment with Labetalol (Means ± S.E.M. n = 10).

Giving separate consideration to the 5 hypertensive subjects with metabolic disorders classifiable as impaired glucose tolerance, the O.G.T.T. curve plotted during treatment with Labetalol, reveals a reduction in glucose and insulin values at the 90th and 120th minute in relation to the values recorded before the administration of the drug. The reduction is statistically significant, however, only for serum insulin, the basal value of which, moreover, seems significantly greater after treatment; the

profile of the insulin curve therefore comes to resemble more closely that of subjects without metabolic disorders. In these same subjects it is not possible to demonstrate significant differences between the glucagon curves plotted before and during treatment (Fig. 6).

In the 5 patients with overt diabetes but not insulin-dependent, the O.G.T.T. curve plotted during treatment, in comparison to the curve plotted before treatment, reveals a constant reduction in the glucose values, although this

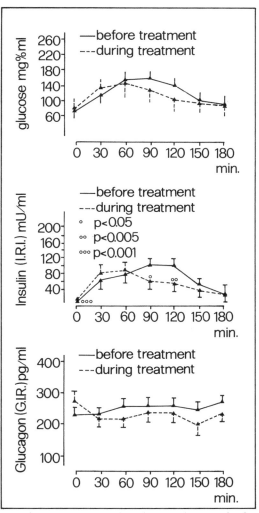

Fig. 6. Serum glucose, insulin and glucagon in the O.G.T.T. curve in hypertensives with reduced carbohydrate tolerance, before treatment and on the 10th day of treatment with Labetalol (Mean ± S.E.M. n = 5).

reduction only appears significant at the 60th minute. Conversely, basal and end-of-curve glucose values overlap. Finally, the glucagon curve shows no difference in relation to the treatment even if, as is usual with diabetic patients, all values found are above the normal range (Fig. 7).

Serum NEFA are reduced in all patients, both diabetic and non-diabetic, during the treatment, even if not to a significant degree (Fig. 8).

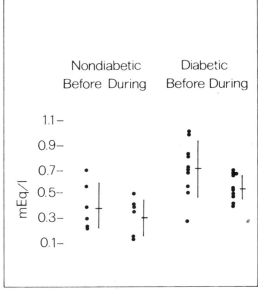

Fig. 8. Plasma levels of NEFA in diabetic and non-diabetic hypertensives, before treatment and on the 10th day of treatment with Labetalol (Mean ± S.E.M. n = 6).

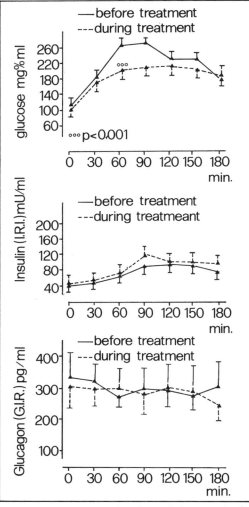

Fig. 7. Serum glucose, insulin and glucagon in the O.G.T.T. curve in hypertensives with clinically overt diabetes, before treatment and on the 10th day of treatment with Labetalol (Mean ±S.E.M. n = 5).

The urinary catecholamines, in both the diabetic and non-diabetic hypertensives, show a considerable increase in statistical significance in their daily excretion during the treatment period (Fig. 9).

However, this increase was not confirmed by the results obtained in the plasma catecholamine assay; in fact, the values of the three fractions (dopamine, adrenalin and noradrenalin), on the contrary, are slightly reduced, and in a non-significant manner, during the administration of Labetalol (Table II).

Discussion

In accordance with the available literature on the subject, our results show that Labetalol, at the doses we used, is an efficacious antihypertensive agent [8, 9, 16, 19, 28]. In fact, systolic and diastolic blood pressure values underwent a constant and statistically significant reduction in all our patients, essential hypertensives of WHO classes I and II.

Heart rate and plasma renin activity are also reduced, but to a moderate and non-signifi-

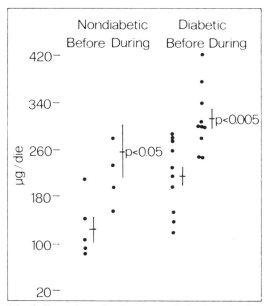

Fig. 9. Excretion of urinary catecholamines in diabetic and non-diabetic hypertensives, before treatment and on the 10th day of treatment with Labetalol (Mean±S.E.M. n = 16).

cant degree. These data, which agree with those reported by other authors [16, 28], we believe may be explained both by considering the peripheral and central haemodynamic effects of the drug and, as far as PRA is concerned, by admitting the simultaneous existence of 2 divergent actions, one being the typically inhibiting action of the beta-blockade and the other a stimulating action attributable to the simultaneous alpha-blocking effect [26, 30].

With regard to the effects of the drug on glucose metabolism, the fact that the glucose, insulin and glucagon curves plotted before and during treatment with Labetalol of non-diabetic hypertensives are virtually identical seems

to us of particular importance. These results, partly confirmed by the limited clinical literature available [1, 19, 23], seem to support the experimental data according to which the simultaneous blockade of the alpha- and beta-receptors at the level of the organs which regulate glucose metabolism, and especially of the receptor system of the insular cells of the pancreas, does not give rise to substantial changes in their endocrinal acitivity either in basal conditions or after stimulus.

Perhaps of greater interest, though without doubt of more difficult interpretation, are our results in subjects affected by impaired glucose tolerance and overt diabetes. In fact, in the group of patients with impaired glucose tolerance we noted, during treatment with Labetalol, a significant increase in serum insulin and its significant reduction at the 90th and 120th minutes, accompanied by a reduction - albeit non-significant - in the glucose levels and no change in the glucagon curve. These data, supported by the findings of Pessina et al., [19] may perhaps be explained by supposing, at the level of the diabetic pancreas, the prevalence of beta-blocking activity over alpha-blocking activity which, by reducing the production of excess insulin tends to give the insulin curve a "normal" profile and thereby favours a better relationship between the insulin and its peripheral receptor.

The group of hypertensives with overt diabetes revealed a decrease in the glucose levels along almost the entire curve profile. This decrease becomes significant at the 60th minute, without any change occurring - in relation to the treatment - in the insulin and glucagon curves. The absence of any change in the insulin curve seems reasonable if it is remembered that the inadequate and delayed insulin re-

Table II. *Plasma catecholamine levels in diabetic and non-diabetic hypertensives, before treatment and on the 10th day of treatment with Labetalol (Mean ± S.E.M. n = 16).*

	DOPAMINE	EPINEPHRINE	NOREPINEPHRINE
BEFORE TREATMENT	58.3±23.5	22.3±5.1	217.5±182.7
DURING TREATMENT	27.7±16.4	17.6±9.0	165.6±90.1

sponse to glucose is characteristic of type II diabetes and of the onset of maturity.

On the other hand, in our results the reduction of the glycemic values during treatment with Labetalol of subjects with overt diabetes, cannot be attributed to any changes in the secretion of glucagon and may therefore, we believe, be explained by two factors: a) reduced neoglycogenesis and glycogenolysis and b) greater influence of the diet followed during the treatment period at the second check in comparison to the pre-treatment check.

As far as the effects of the drug on glucagon secretion are concerned, the absence of any significant difference as a result of the treatment, in both the diabetic and non-diabetic subjects examined, would seem to confirm the existence, even at the level of the insular alpha cells, of a double receptor system with a divergent effect. On the other hand, our patients did not experience such excursions in their insulin and glucose levels as to bring about a reflex variation in the secretion of glucagon [2].

In order to document, in the metabolic effect of the drug, the possible influence of extra-pancreatic factors such as the catecholamines - which various authors [11, 13] have found, using the fluorometric method, at increased levels in both the blood and the urine during treatment with Labetalol - during the course of our study we carried out an assay of the daily excretion of urinary catecholamines by means of the fluorometric method and of the basal plasma catecholamines by the radioenzymic method. According to our results, a significant increase in the urinary catecholaminis is reflected in a slight, non-significant lowering of basal plasma catecholamine levels, of dopamine as well as of epinephrine and norepinephrine.

This finding, comparable to those reached by other authors [2, 13, 15, 18] using certain betablockers and to the results reported by Hamilton [11] using Labetalol, would seem to permit us to exclude any real increase in the circulating catecholamines and lead us to believe that the presumed increase found by other authors using the fluorometric and spectrophotometric methods, is to be attributed rather to an interference of the Labetalol metabolites in the above-mentioned assay methods.

This observation, furthermore, seems to be confirmed in our study by the slight decrease noted during treatment of the circulating NEFA. This reduction, of no statistical importance, confirmed by recent publications [10, 14] containing similar observations with various beta-blocking drugs, is not, however, such as to lend plausibility to the hypothesis that the reductions in the glucose values found in the O.G.T.T. curves of diabetic subjects may be attributed to it.

It is our belief, therefore, that the results of our investigation permit us to conclude that oral treatment with Labetalol does not, at least with short-term use, alter the carbohydrate tolerance and the insulin response of subjects without metabolic disorders, whereas in diabetic subjects whether with impaired glucose tolerance or with overt diabetes, serum insulin and glucose changes have no apparent clinical importance.

Drug therapy of systemic arterial hypertension is still mainly based on trial and error, the only criterium of efficacy, in general, being the degree of blood-pressure reduction achieved. It is evident that lowering of blood presure to preferably normal levels must remain the prime concern of physicans; it is, however, also obvious that, ideally, anti-hypertensive treatment should not only aim at lowering systemic blood pressure, but should achieve this by reversing the pathophysiological changes induced by the disease process. That implies, of course, that, in choosing an anti-hypertensive agent, factors such as age of the subject and stage of the disease, and the pharmacological profile of the drug have to be taken into account. Since hypertension is primarily a circulatory disorder prompting above all cardiovascular changes and often morbid cardiovascular events, haemodynamic aspects must reasonably play a cardinal rôle in all therapeutical considerations.

The purpose of this paper is to briefly review the haemodynamic consequences of adrenoceptor blockade in hypertensive patients; since different haemodynamic patterns, however, are seen in the course of hypertension a short review of its natural history in terms of haemodynamics is given as well.

The haemodynamic pattern of hypertension

Irrespective of which causative mechanisms may eventually be involved in the multifactorial disorder called essential hypertension, it is axiomatic that such mechanisms would have to influence blood pressure through changes in cardiac output or in systemic vascular resistance, or in both of these variables. During the last 15 years it has become evident that their mutual importance in generating high blood pressure differs depending upon the age of the subject and the stage of the hypertensive disorder [5, 15, 17, 18].

Early essential hypertension

In younger subjects (18 to 29 years) with mild essential hypertension, cardiac output at rest is usually higher than in normotensive age-matched controls; stroke volume is usually normal; heart rate is increased. Total systemic vascular resistance, however, is within normal limits.

This increased cardiac output in early essential hypertension is often referred to as a "hyperkinetic" circulation. However, the observation that oxygen uptake is also increased indicates that the rise in cardiac output corresponds to an increase in metabolic rate. The cause of this abnormality is unknown; it might be related to increased sympathetic activity which has been shown to exist in hypertensives at this stage compared with age-matched controls [11, 12] (Fig. 1). During exercise a different haemodynamic pattern is seen: cardiac output is no longer high, but rather subnormal. During maximal exercise it is significantly lower than in age-matched controls when related to oxygen uptake. Surprisingly enough, stroke volume is lower than in age-matched controls. This is partly compensated for by an increased heart rate, but the compensation falls short during strenuous exercise. Furthermore, total systemic resistance during exercise does not fall to the levels seen in normotensive controls.

Thus, already in subjects with mild WHO stage I essential hypertension, some kind of left ventricular function disturbance as well as alterations in vascular resistance are present; they are reflected in a subnormal stroke volume during exercise and by a lower degree of exercise-induced vasodilation [15].

Established hypertension

In subjects older than 30 years with mild-to-moderate established hypertension (WHO stages I and II), cardiac output at rest is usually normal; total systemic resistance is increased. During exercise cardiac output becomes subnormal, even at lower levels of activity, and is associated with a subnormal stroke volume and high heart rate. The arteriovenous oxygen difference is increased. Total systemic resistance is significantly raised both at rest and during exercise.

References

1. Andersson O., Berglund G., Hansson L.: Antihypertensive action, time of onset and effects on carbohydrate metabolism of labetalol. *Brit. J. Clin. Pharmacol.* Suppl. 757-761, 1976.
2. Bengt-Göran Hansson, Bernt Hökfelt: The effect of sympathetic inhibition on plasma levels of catecholamines, growth hormone, glucagon and cortisol. *Acta Med. Scand.* Suppl. 628, "Symposium et Foresta" Stockholm, 2 June 1978.
3. Cerasi E., Luft R., Efendic S.: Effect of adrenergic blocking agents on insulin response to glucose infusion in man. *Acta Endocrinol.* 69, 335, 1972.
4. Colwell S.A.: Inhibition of insulin secretion by catecholamines in pheochromocytoma. *Ann. Intern. Med.* 71: 251, 1969.
5. Cryer P.E., Herman C.M., Sode: Insulin release during alpha-adrenergic receptor blockade: primacy of the glycemic stimulus. *Endocrinology* 89, 918, 1971.
6. Day J.L., Simpson N., Metcalfe J., Page R.L.: Metabolic consequences of atenolol and propranolol in treatment of essential hypertension. *Brit. Med. J.* 1, 77-80, 1979.
7. Ekberg G., Bengt-Göran Hansson: Glucose tolerance and insulin release in hypertensive patients treated with cardioselective beta-receptor blocking agent: metoprolol. *Acta Med. Scand.* 202, 393-397, 1977.
8. Flammer J.: Cardiovascular and endocrine profile of adrenergic neurone blockade in normal and hypertensive man. *Am. J. Med.* 66, 34-42, 1979.
9. Frishman W.: Clinical pharmacology of the new beta-adrenergic blocking drugs. Part 7. New horizons in beta-adrenoreceptor blockade therapy: Labetalol. *Am. Heart J.* 98, 5, 660-665, 1979.

10. Gagliardino J., Bellone C., Doria J., Sanchez J., Pereyra V.: Adrenergic regulation of basal serum glucose, NEFA, and insulin levels. *Horm. Metab. Res.* 2, 318, 1970.

11. Hamilton C.A., Jones D.H., Dargie H.J., Reid J.L.: Does Labetalol increase excretion of urinary catecholamines? *Brit. Med. J.* 16, 800, 1978.

12. Hendrika J., Waal-Manning: Metabolic effects of beta-adrenoreceptor blockers. *Drugs* 11, 121, 1976.

13. Hansson B.G.: Long-term non-selective and cardioselective beta-receptor blockade in hypertensive patients. Effects on circulatory parameters, catecholamines and renin activity under basal conditions and in connection with exercise and hypoglycemia. *Acta Med. Scand.* Suppl. 598, 1976.

14. Hiroo Imura, Yuzuru Kato, Masaki Ikeda, Masachika Morimoto, Mikio Yawata: Effect of adrenergic-blocking or stimulating agents on plasma growth hormone, immunoreactive insuline, and blood free fatty acid levels in man. *J. Clin. Invest.* 50, 1069-1079, 1971.

15. Jones D.H.: Plasma noradrenaline concentration in essential hypertension during long-term beta-adrenoceptor blockade with oxprenolol. *Brit. J. Clin. Pharmacol.* 9, 27, 1980.

16. Jockes A.M.: Acute haemodynamic effects of labetalol and its subsequent use as an oral hypotensive agent. *Brit. J. Clin. Pharmacol.* Suppl. 789-793, 1976.

17. Lager I., Smith U., Blöhmé G.: Effect of cardioselective and non-selective beta-blockade on the hypoglycaemic response in insulin-dependent diabetics. *Lancet*, 1, 458-462, 1979.

18. Lijueu P.J., Amery A.K., Fagard R.M., Reybronck T.M.: The effects of beta-adrenoceptor blockade on renin, angiotensin, aldosterone and catecholamines at rest and during exercise. *Brit. J. Clin. Pharmacol.* 7, 175, 1979.

19. Pessina A., Pagnan A., Hlede M., Sarti F., Guarin P., Palatini A., Semplicini A., Dal Palù C.: Azione antiipertensiva ed effetti metabolici del labetalolo. pp. 200-207. In: *Atti Conv. Int. Ipertensione: Nuove prospettive terapeutiche.* Venezia, 18-20 maggio 1978. Glaxo Italia 1978, 269.

20. Persson I., Lars Larsen: Serum insulin concentration after alpha-adrenergic blockade and secretion in diabetics. *Acta Endocrinol.* 71, 331, 1972.

21. Porte D. Jr.: Beta-adrenergic stimulation of insulin release in man. *Diabetes* 16, 150, 1967.

22. Porte D. Jr., Graber A.L., Kuzuya T., Williams R.H.: The effect of epinephrine on immunoreactive insulin levels in man *J. Clin. Invest.* 45, 228, 1966.

23. Petralito A., Lunetta M., Mangiafico R.A., Liuzzo A., Fiore C.E.: Effetti del labetalolo sul metabolismo glicidico in soggetti ipertesi. *Boll. Soc. Ital. Card.* 509, 1979.

24. Robertson R.P., Porte D.: Adrenergic modulation of basal insulin secretion in man. *Diabetes* 22, 1, 1973.

25. Vance S.E., Buchanan K.D., O'Hara D., Williams R.H., Porte D.: Insulin and glucagon response in subjects with pheochromocytoma: effect of alpha-adrenergic blockade. *J. Clin. Endocrinol.* 29, 911, 1969.

26. Vandongen R.: The inhibition of renin secretion by alpha-adrenergic stimulation in the isolated rat kidney. *Clin. Sci. Mol. Med.* 47, 471, 1974.

27. Waal-Manning H.J.,: Metabolic effect of beta-adrenoreceptor blockers. *Drugs*, 11 Suppl. 1, 121-126, 1976.

28. Weidmann P.: Alpha and beta-adrenergic blockade with orally administered labetalol in hypertension. *Am. J. Cardiol.* 41, 570-576, 1978.

29. William-Olsson T., Fellenius E., Björntorp P., Smith U.: Differences in metabolic responses to beta-adrenergic stimulation after propranolol and metoprolol administration. *Acta Med. Scand.* 205, 201-206, 1979.

30. Zanchetti A.S.: Neural regulation of renin release, Experimental evidence and clinical implications in arterial hypertension. *Circulation* 56, 5, 691, 1977.

Hypertension, recent advances and research
edited by M. Condorelli, A. Zanchetti
Cortina International, Verona 1982

Relationship between arterial hypertension and intralymphocytic sodium concentration

F.V. COSTA, E. AMBROSIONI, L. MONTEBUGNOLI, F. TARTAGNI, B. MAGNANI

Department of Cardiology and Department of Clinical Pharmacology, University of Bologna, Italy

Key words. Arterial Hypertension; Intralymphocytic Sodium Content; Ion Transport; Sodium; Lymphocytes; Stabilized Essential Hypertension; Non-stabilized Essential Hypertension; Sodium Metabolism Defect; Low-sodium Diet; Familial High Blood Pressure; Captopril; Anti-hypertensive Drugs.

Summary. In the course of the last few years a number of studies have stressed the existence of an alteration of ion transport at cell membrane level in patients suffering from arterial hypertension. The study of intralymphocytic sodium content (ILSC) has provided further confirmation of this hypothesis and has laid stress on the following points.
The ILSC in patients with essential hypertension (EH) is always higher than that recorded in normotensive subjects provided the latter have no family history of hypertension. In the secondary forms (with the exception of Conn's disease) the ILSC values are normal.
There is a total overlap between the ILSC values recorded in adults and those recorded in children, just as there are no differences in the percentages obtained in subjects who, in the various subgroups examined, present ILSC values higher than the norm.
In subjects with stabilized essential hypertension, there exists a correlation between ILSC and diastolic and mean BP.
The incubation of lymphocytes from normotensive subjects in plasma from essential hypertensive subjects induces an increase in ILSC to above normal values.
Such an increase may also be induced by digitalis glycosides.
In subjects with non-stabilized hypertension, the response to adrenergic stimuli is much greater, in terms of the rise in diastolic BP, in subjects with high ILSC.
A low-sodium diet brings about a marked reduction in ILSC only in subjects with non-stabilized hypertension and not in normotensive subjects nor in subjects with stabilized hypertension.
In the course of anti-hypertensive treatment, only diuretics and Captopril bring about a reduction in ILSC.
Taken as a whole, the data gathered enable us to formulate a number of hypotheses:
A sodium metabolism defect exists in essential hypertension patients, which would appear to be present as early as in infancy and which enables us to identify subjects "at risk" (normotensive subjects with family positivity and high ILSC, non-stabilized hypertensive subjects with high ILSC).
This defect would appear to be bound up with the existence of a plasma factor which would not seem to be present in secondary hypertension.
A low-sodium diet in subjects with non-stabilized hypertension reduces not only ILSC but also BP. Whether it is capable of definitively blocking the development of stable essential hypertension is something which we will find out only on the basis of a lengthy follow-up period.
ILSC enables us to identify, within the non-stabilized hypertensive group, those subjects with a higher degree of reactivity to adrenergic stimuli.
Furthermore, ILSC provides us with useful data with regard to the action mechanisms of anti-hypertensive drugs.

Many studies during recent years have demonstrated an impairment of intracellular sodium metabolism in patients with essential hypertension (EH) [1, 2, 3]. More recent data have shown that the abnormal net Na^+ and K^+ fluxes in erythrocytes of patients with EH can result in intracellular Na^+ (and Ca_2^+) retention leading to high blood pressure (HBP) [4].

The defect seems to be due to a Na^+/K^+ cotransport defect which is present also in 50% of normotensive children born of one hypertensive parent, while, in the case of children born of two hypertensive parents, the abnormality is more frequent [5]. All these observations seem to indicate that EH is a genetically predetermined disease whose development could be caused by environmental factors such as dietary salt intake, stress, etc. Nevertheless, data on erythrocytes are qualitative and not quantitative and, in the case of leucocytes there is an overlapping between values of normotensives and hypertensives [6]. A few years ago we described a method for the determination of intralymphocytic sodium concentration (ILSC) by which we can clearly differentiate normotensives from people with EH [7, 8] as is shown in Table I. Among normotensives, subjects with family history of HBP have mean values greater than normotensives without familial HBP, and 69.2% of these subjects have abnormally high ILSC values (26 nMol/Kg). In people with non-stabilized HBP (we defined as non-stabilized or borderline hypertensives those subjects who exhibited at least one BP recording out of three above 140 mmHg systolic or 90 mmHg diastolic and at least one measurement below 140/90 mmHg) the percentage with high ILSC values is 58.3%. In the case of stable EH 100% of patients have ILSC values greater then 26 nMol/Kg. Looking at children under 12 years of age we found mean ILSC values and percentages of subjects with high ILSC which do not differ from adults. This observation suggests that ILSC values are stable during lifetime and that the NA^+/K^+ transport defect is inherited and genetically predetermined. No difference can be found between males and females or between age groups.

Another important observation emerged from our data: ILSC in the case of secondary forms of HBP is normal except in the case of Conn's disease (Table II). This provides further evidence for the hypothesis of a genetically pre-determined disease; this hypothesis was confirmed by experiments of cross-incubation.

When lymphocytes of normotensives are

Table I. *ILSC values (mean + s. dev.) in normotensives, borderline and hypertensives.*

	NORMAL BP (F−)	NORMAL BP (F+)	BORDERLINE	ESSENTIAL HBP
CHILDREN (age 8-12)	22.2 ± 2.8 (24)	28.3 ± 4.7 (24)	26.6 ± 5.3 (26)	30.0 ± 0.9 (2)
% with ILSC > 26 mmol/Kg	0	66.6	50	100
ADULTS (age 24-70)	21.9 ± 3.1 (40)	27.9 ± 4.2 (26)	27.2 ± 5.6 (84)	33.2 ± 3.1 (81)
% with ILSC > 26 mmol/Kg	0	69.2	58.3	100

F− = No history of familial hypertension.
F+ = history of familial hypertension.
( ) = No. of subjects.

Table II. *ILSC values (mean ± S.D.) in secundary hypertension.*

RENO-VASCULAR (3 cases)	22.1 ± 3.7 mmol/Kg
RENO-PARENCHIMAL (9 cases)	22.4 ± 3.1 mmol/Kg
PHEOCHROMOCYTOMA (2 cases)	21.2 ± 1.8 mmol/Kg
PRIMARY ALDOSTERONISM (2 cases)	36.9 ± 5.6 mmol/Kg

incubated in plasma of patients with EH (Table III) ILSC increases from 23.8 ± 3 mMol/Kg to 37.1 ± 4 nMol/Kg while incubating lymphocytes of patients with EH in plasma of other hypertensives or of people with normal BP does not cause any change. This phenomenon seems to confirm the hypothesis of the existence of a plasmatic factor, the so-called "natriuretic factor" [9] which inhibits the Na^+/K^+ pump

in patients with EH. This factor seems not to be present in secondary forms of hypertension where ILSC is normal. A similar increase of ILSC can be induced by incubating for 60 min. lymphocytes with ouabain (20 ug/ml), a substance which inhibits the Na^+/K^+ pump (Table IV). Both in the case of normotensives and patients with EH we observed a significant increase in ILSC whose values after incubation with ouabain are similar in normotensives and in hypertensives. This increase is self-limiting, probably because of the action of some ouabain-independent mechanism.

We also observed that ILSC values significantly correlate with systolic BP ($r = 0.31$; $P < 0.005$) and diastolic BP ($r = 0.58$; $P < 0.001$)) in patients with EH while this correlation is not detectable in the case of normotensives or in patients with secondary HBP. In the studies regarding erythrocytes and leucocytes no correlation between intracellular Na^+ concentration and BP was reported and this lack of correla-

Table III. *Variations of ILSC of normotensives without familial hypertension incubated in plasma of essential hypertensives (above) and of people with essential hypertension incubated in plasma of normotensives (below) without familial hypertension (mean values ± S.D. expressed in mmol/Kg).*

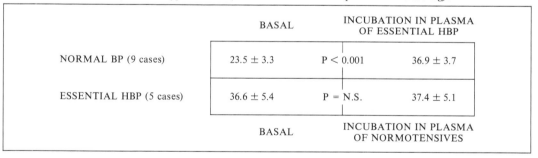

	BASAL		INCUBATION IN PLASMA OF ESSENTIAL HBP
NORMAL BP (9 cases)	23.5 ± 3.3	P < 0.001	36.9 ± 3.7
ESSENTIAL HBP (5 cases)	36.6 ± 5.4	P = N.S.	37.4 ± 5.1
	BASAL		INCUBATION IN PLASMA OF NORMOTENSIVES

Table IV. *Variation of ILSC in normotensives and essential hypertensives incubated in homologous plasma added with 20 µg of ouabain (mean values ± S.D. expressed in mmol/Kg/wet weight).*

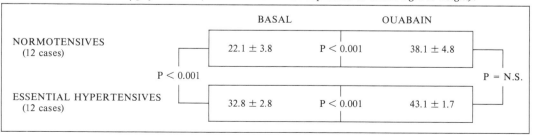

		BASAL		OUABAIN	
NORMOTENSIVES (12 cases)		22.1 ± 3.8	P < 0.001	38.1 ± 4.8	
	P < 0.001				P = N.S.
ESSENTIAL HYPERTENSIVES (12 cases)		32.8 ± 2.8	P < 0.001	43.1 ± 1.7	

tion may be due to the fact that these cells do not represent a good model for the intracellular compartment (most of all for the muscular cells of the arterial wall).

Our results suggest that our model is a good one for the investigation about what is happening in the wall of peripheral arteries. In fact, some studies have suggested [9,10] that the increase in peripheral vascular resistances which is a typical feature of EH is caused by an increase in intracellular Na^+ (and consequently in Ca_2^+). This increase causes an enhancement of vascular reactivity and a rise in BP.

Another very important field of investigation is non-stabilized (or borderline) hypertension. We determined ILSC concentrations in a group of 111 young people (ages 8-35 years) with non stabilized hypertension and we found (Table V) that the values are widely dispersed between normal and high values and with a mean value which is halfway between normotensive and essential hypertensive ILSC values. This large dispersion of ILSC probably reflects the presence in this group of very different subjects, part of whom will become hypertensive and part of whom probably will never develop stable HBP. Up to now a test to identify non-stabilized hypertensives with high risk of becoming stable hypertensives is not available. This is a big problem because we do not know if these subjects have to be treated or not. It is evident that EH begins to develop early in life and that both genetic and environmental factors are involved. At present we are not sure that ILSC is a good marker for detecting non-stabilized hypertensives at risk but we have tried to better define some aspects assessing the behaviour of some parameters during tests of adrenergic stimulation and during a low-salt diet. It has been observed that [11] tests such as mental arithmetic can induce a greater increase in BP in non-stabilized hypertensives and in normotensives with familial hypertension than in normotensives with no history of familial hypertension and that this greater response can be further enhanced by high sodium intake [12]. We tried to detect if it is possible to relate the response to mental arithmetic to ILSC values in borderline hypertension. We noted (Fig. 1) a significantly greater increase in DBP in borderline subjects when compared to normal people, but if we separately consider borderline subjects with normal (≤ 26 mMol/Kg) and high (> 26 mMol/Kg) ILSC values we find that the increase is much greater in people with high ILSC, while if ILSC is normal there is no significant difference between normotensives and borderline subjects. Another very interesting observation derived from this study is that such a different response is not detectable if we consider SBP and HR. The increase in ILSC seems thus to affect the response of peripheral vascular resistances and does not affect cardiac output. A long-term follow-up will tell us if borderline people with a greater response to mental stress and high ILSC values will become stable hypertensives.

We also observed that [13] dietary salt restriction in non-stabilized hypertensives induces a significant reduction in both BP and ILSC (Table VI). This reduction disappears completely when a normal salt diet is started again. Normal subjects and patients with stable HBP do not show this phenomenon. Perhaps, in the case of stable HBP a longer period of sodium restriction is needed to obtain a modification of ILSC. Among anti-hypertensive drugs only diuretic agents induced a significant decrease in ILSC, while using methyldopa, clonidine,

Table V. *ILSC values in patients with borderline hypertension without (FAM−) and with (FAM+) family history of hypertension.*

	ILSC mmol/Kg (mean ± S.D.)	
TOTAL N. 111 cases	27.0 ± 5.0	
		P = N.S.
FAM− N. 47 cases	27.8 ± 5.3	
		P = N.S.
FAM+ N. 64 cases	26.4 ± 5.6	

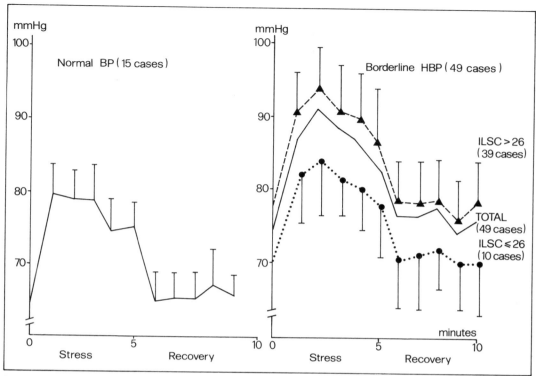

Fig. 1. Variations of diastolic BP during stress (mental arithmetic) in normal people without familial hypertension (left) and in people with borderline hypertension (right). (ILSC values are expressed in mmol/Kg wet weight).

Table VI. *Effects of dietary sodium intake on ILSC in people with normal BP, labile HBP and stable essential HBP (ILSC values are expressed in mmol/Kg/wet weight).*

	Basal	Low-salt diet (3 months)	Normal salt diet (2 months)
NORMAL BP	22.3 ± 2.4	22.5 ± 2.9	
LABILE HBP	31.6 ± 3.4	24.5 ± 3.1	30.9 ± 2.8
STABLE HBP	34.6 ± 2.1	34.0 +	

Table VII. *Effects of treatment with Captopril on ILSC and blood pressure.*

PATIENT	BP mmHg		ILSC mmol/Kg	
	PRE	CPT	PRE	CPT
1	210/160	170/90	39.5	27.1
2	180/110	110/95	33.7	25.1
3	195/130	140/110	35.5	27.3
4	195/130	160/100	30.7	23.4
5	170/130	150/100	36.0	29.5
6	190/115	175/110	35.0	31.8
7	170/110	135/90	41.0	26.5
8	130/110	105/85	30.0	24.2
9	220/135	130/95	30.6	25.5

CPT = Captopril 150 mg T.I.D.

betablockers and guanethidine no variation was observed [13].

A very interesting observation was made during chronic therapy with captopril (Table VII). In all cases in which a reduction in ILSC was observed it was accompanied by a decrease in BP. The only patient in which we did not observe a significant reduction in BP did not show a reduction in ILSC. This phenomenon seems to indicate that captopril somehow exerts an action upon the NA^+/K^+ pump; this action could be related to an inhibition of aldosterone and could explain, at any rate partially, the anti-hypertensive action of this drug whose inhibition of the angiotensin-converting enzyme seems to be not the only mechanism of action [14]. All the observations, rather than giving definite answers, open up a new series of questions but as of now we can state the following points:

— ILSC values correlate with BP values in patients with EH;

— ILSC is high in EH and in a high percentage of normotensives with familial hypertension;

— ILSC values are similar in adults and children; this supports the hypothesis that EH is a genetically predetermined disease;

— ILSC is a good parameter for identifying people with borderline HBP with exaggerated response to stress;

— a low salt diet can normalize BP and ILSC in borderline patients;

— the Na^+/K^+ pump defect seems to be related to a circulating factor which is present in EH but not in secondary forms of hypertension.

References

1. Postnov, Y.V., Orlov, S.N., Gulax, J V., Shevenko, A.S.: Evidence of altered permeabi of the erythrocyte membrane for sodium and potassium ions in spontaneously hypertensive rats. *Clin. Sci. Mol. Med.,* 51, 169-172, 1976.

2. Edmondson, R.P.S., Thomas, R. D., Hilton, P. S., Patrick, J., Jones, F.S.: Abnormal leucocyte composition and sodium transport in essential hypertension. *Lancet*, 2, 1003-1005, 1975.

3. Garay, R., Meyer, P.: A new test showing abnormal net Na^+ and K^+ fluxes in erythrocytes of essential hypertensive patients. *Lancet*, 1, 349-353, 1979.

4. Reuter, H., Blaunstein, M.P., Haeusler, G.: Na^+-Ca^{++} exchange and tension development in arterial smooth muscle. Philosophical Transaction of the Royal Society of London; *Bio. Sci.*, B 265, 87-89, 1973.

5. Garay, R.P., Dagher, G., Meyer, P.: An inherited Na^+, K^+ cotransport defect in essential hypertension. *7th Meeting of the International Society of Hypertension* (Abstract), 39, 1980.

6. Araoye, M.A., Khatry, I.M., Yao, L.L., Freis, E.D.: Leucocyte intracellular cations in hypertension; effects of anti-hypertensive drugs. *Am. Heart J.*, 96, 731-738, 1978.

7. Tartagni, F., Ambrosioni, E., Montebugnoli, L., Magnani, B.: Nuovo metodo per la determinazione del sodio intralinfocitario. *G. Clin. Med.*, 60, 500-506, 1979.

8. Ambrosioni, E., Tartagni, F., Montebugnoli, L., Magnani, B.: Intralymphocytic sodium in hypertensive patients: a significant correlation. *Clin. Sci.*, 57, 325s-327s, 1979.

9. Overbeck, H.W., Pamnani, M.B., Akera, T., Brody, T.M., Haddy, F.J.: Depressed function of a ouabain-sensitive sodium potassium pump in blood vessels from renal hypertensive dogs. *Circ. Res.*, 38 suppl II, 48-52, 1976.

10. Tobian, L.: Interrelationship of electrolytes, juxtaglomerular cells and hypertension. *Physiol. Rev.*, 40, 280-312, 1960.

11. Falkner, B., Onesti, G., Angelakos, E.T., Fernandes, M., Langman, C.: Cardiovascular response to mental stress in normal adolescents with hypertensive parents. *Hypertension*, 1, 23-30, 1979.

12. Falkner, B., Onesti, G., Gould, A.: Effect of salt loading on cardiovascular response to mental stress in adolescents. *7th Meeting of the International Society of Hypertension (Abstract)*, 31, 1980.

13. Ambrosioni, E., Costa, F.V., Montebugnoli, L., Magnani, B.: Effects of antihypertensive therapy on intralymphocytic sodium content. *Drugs Expt. Clin. Res.*, (in press).

14. Gavras, H., Brunner, H.R. Turini, G.R., Kershaw, C.P., Tifft, S., Cuttelod, I, Gavras, R.A., Vukovich, R. and McKinstry, D.N.: Antihypertensive effect of the oral angiotensin-converting enzyme inhibitor SQ 14 225 in man. *New Engl. J. Med.*, 298, 991-995, 1977.

Hypertension, recent advances and research
edited by M. Condorelli, A. Zanchetti
Cortina International, Verona 1982

The influence of Labetalol on the haemodynamic parameters related to the oxygen consumption of the myocardium in hypertensive and anginal subjects

A. CHERCHI

Department of Cardiovascular Pathology, University of Cagliari, Italy.

Key words. Labetalol; Haemodynamic Parameters; Hypertension; Angina Pectoris; Myocardial Oxygen Consumption; Chlorthalidone; Placebo; Trinitroglycerin; Double Product HR x SP; Triple Product HR x SP x LVET.

Summary. The action of Labetalol on the main haemodynamic parameters related to the oxygen consumption of the myocardium, the double product $HR \times SP$ and the triple product $HR \times SP \times LVET$ were studied in hypertensive patients and in patients with angina due to strain.
In 6 patients - WHO Classes I and II - the acute intravenous administration of 50 mg of Labetalol brought about a significant decrease in systolic BP, diastolic BP, HR and the double product during exercise.
In a further 8 hypertensives - WHO Classes I and II - the administration of 150-600 mg/day of Labetalol for 21 days caused a significant reduction during exercise in systolic and diastolic BP, HR, double product and triple product, without altering work capacity.
Finally, in 6 non-hypertensive patients suffering from angina due to strain, Labetalol significantly decreased ischaemic electrical phenomena and angina symptoms, whilst at the same time reducing the double and triple products.

Introduction

Labetalol is the only drug to date which has both alpha- and beta-blocking properties. In other words, it combines the action proper to adrenergic beta-blockers with action related to concomitant adrenergic alpha-blocking activity [1-2].

It was therefore probable that Labetalol was capable of reducing the oxygen consumption of the myocardium considerably thanks to the combined central bradycardiac action of the beta-blockade and the peripheral vaso-dilatory action of the alpha-blockade.

This study summarizes the results obtained in non-anginal hypertensives, comparing Labetalol with Propranolol, on the one hand, and with Chlorthalidone, on the other hand, and in anginal non-hypertensives, comparing the effect of Labetalol with that of TNG on the haemodynamic parameters most closely related to the oxygen consumption of the myocardium, especially the product of Heart Rate $\times$ Systolic Peak.

Effect of the acute administration of Labetalol on the double product HR $\times$ SP at rest and during exercise in hypertensive patients. Comparison with placebo and with Propranolol.

Patients and Method

Six male hypertensives, average age 39 ± 4 years, WHO classes I and II, were studied at rest and during exercise to assess the effect of the intravenous administration of 50 mg of Labetalol or 10 mg of Propranolol under double-blind conditions [3].

The response to the drugs was studied at rest in both the supine and sitting positions, and during muscular exercise steadily increasing at a rate of 10 watts/min. on the cycloergometer until exhaustion, according to our normal laboratory procedures [4, 5, 6]. Muscular exercise in the sitting position on Lanooy's hyperbolic cycloergometer, increasing steadily, at the rate of 10 watts per minute until exhaustion or the appearance of other symptoms, such as angina, intense dyspnea, etc. [4, 5].

The systolic time intervals were calculated using Weissler's method [6] by recording, in addition to the electrocardiogram, also the phonocardiogram with the aid of a special microphone held in the apex position by a strip of rubber, and the carotidogram (ususally the right), by means of a transducer held in place by a special collar [6, 7].

In our study, the electrocardiograms and the STIs, were obtained using a Siemens Elema 6-channel Mingograf.

The tests were randomized using Latin squares and carried out on successive days.

The statistical analysis was effected using Student's t test for paired data.

Results

The double product HR $\times$ SP (Fig. 1) was lower after Labetalol in comparison with placebo in the supine rest position, during muscular exercise and recovery, with no significant differences in comparison with Propranolol.

However, there is no overlapping of the action mechanism of the two drugs. In fact, systolic BP (Fig. 2) was reduced by Labetalol, in comparison with placebo, in the sitting and lying positions, during exercise and recovery, with no significant difference in comparison with Propranolol which, however, had not modified systolic BP during rest.

Labetalol significantly lowered diastolic BP (Fig. 2), especially during muscular exercise, as compared to both placebo and Propranolol.

HR (Fig. 3) was reduced to a significant extent by Propranolol in all three circumstances:

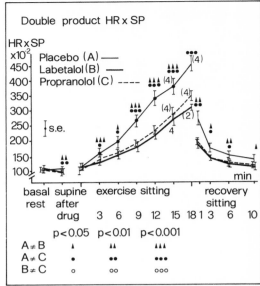

Fig. 1. Evaluation of the product of Heart Rate $\times$ Systolic Pressure after placebo, Labetalol and Propranolol in relation to different experimental times: during rest in the supine position, in basal conditions and 3 minutes after the injection of the different drugs, during rest after sitting on the cycloergometer for 3 minutes (0), during muscular exercise at progressive increases of 10 watts/min. until exhaustion, and during recovery, still in the sitting position on the cycloergometer.

rest, exercise and recovery, whereas the action of Labetalol was significant only in the latter two, i.e. during exercise and recovery.

To summarize, Labetalol administered intravenously to hypertensive patients proved capable of reducing the double product of HR $\times$ SP at rest, during exercise and recovery, significantly in comparison with placebo and in like measure in comparison with Propranolol, at the same time as significantly lowering systolic BP and - unlike Propranolol - also diastolic BP.

Effect of the medium-term administration of Labetalol on the double product HR $\times$ SP and on the triple product HR $\times$ SP $\times$ LVET at rest, during exercise and after medium-term administration. Comparison with Chlorthalidone

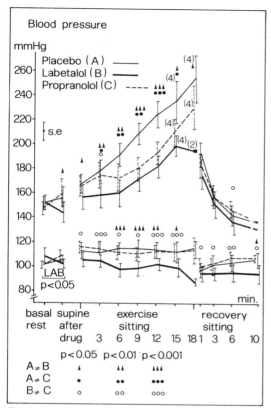

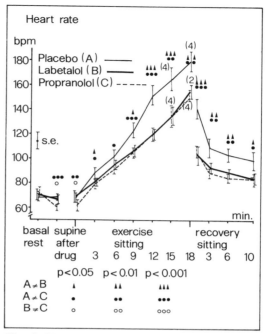

Fig. 3. Heart Rate trend after placebo, Labetalol and Propranolol in relation to the various experimental times. (See Fig. 1).

Fig. 2. Trends in systolic blood pressure (top graph) and diastolic blood pressure (bottom graph) after placebo, Labetalol, and Propranolol at the different experimental times. (See Fig. 1).

Patients and Method

The patients studied were 8 male hypertensives, average age 40 ± 2 years, WHO Classes I and II; the patients, whose informed consent was obtained, were volunteers in the context of an experiment carried out under double-blind conditions [8].

Each patient constituted his own control.

The patients were studied at rest and during muscular exercise with progressive 10 watt/min. increases until exhaustion, according to the above-described method, at the beginning of the experiment (control) and after two courses of therapy each lasting 21 days, with the two sequences - Chlorthalidone-Labetalol and Labetalol-Chlorthalidone - randomized.

The statistical calculation was effected using Student's t test for paired data as between the two drugs and the control.

After 21 days of treatment with Labetalol (150-600 mg/day) and with Chlorthalidone (50-100 mg/day) systolic and diastolic BP proved to be significantly reduced (Fig. 6).

The double product HR × SP (Fig. 4) was reduced, in relation to the pre-treatment control, by Labetalol during rest, exercise and recovery, especially at the heaviest loads ad during recovery even as compared to Chlorthalidone.

The triple product HR × SP × LVET (Fig. 5) was likewise reduced after Labetalol, though there was no significant difference in the values obtained during rest or exercise in comparison with Chlorthalidone.

The action mechanisms of the two drugs do not overlap, however; in fact, Labetalol significantly reduced systolic and diastolic BP du-

41

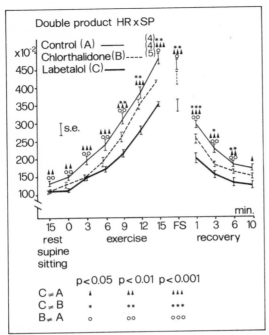

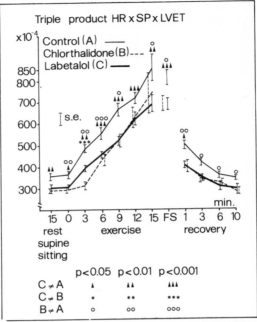

Fig. 4. Behaviour of the product HR × SP during rest (supine and sitting), during progressively increasing muscular exercise and during recovery, in control conditions and after the oral administration of Chlorthalidone (50-100 mg/day) and Labetalol (150-600 mg/day). Labetalol and Chlorthalidone both brought about a significant decrease in the double product during rest, exercise and recovery; however, Labetalol has a more marked activity than Chlorthalidone during the more intense exercise and during recovery.

Fig. 5. Behaviour of the triple product HR × SP × LVET in the same experimental conditions as described in Fig. 4. Labetalol and Chlorthalidone significantly reduce the triple product without significant differences.

Effect of Labetalol on both the double and triple product during rest and muscular exercise in patients suffering from angina. Comparison with placebo and trinitroglycerin.

Patients and Method

ring rest (Fig. 6) and during exercise, to a degree not dissimilar to the effect of Chlorthalidone, but heart rate (Fig. 7) was lowered during rest and exercise only by Labetalol.

The greater effect of Chlorthalidone on the triple product as compared to the double product is due to the reduction in LVET caused by the diuretic.

To sum up, the chronic administration of Labetalol, besides significantly lowering BP, also brings about a significant reduction in the double and triple products, parameters notoriously related to the oxygen consumption of the myocardium, during both rest and muscular exercise.

The patients studied were all suffering from angina due to typical strain and whose condition had been stable for at least 3 months. Their electrocardiograms before treatment were normal and they showed the usual RS-T modifications of an ischaemic nature during muscular exercise [9].

All patients, males aged 51 ± 4 years, were volunteers and fully informed.

The trial was carried out on three successive days in the morning at least one hour after light carbohydrate ingestion, comparing the effect of Labetalol (50 mg i.v.), with a drug of known action (TNG 0.35 mg i.v.) and with placebo (physiological solution 10 ml i.v.).

The trial was performed in double-blind

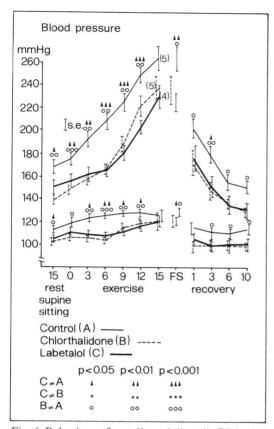

Control (A) ——
Chlorthalidone (B) -----
Labetalol (C) ——

	p<0.05	p<0.01	p<0.001
C≠A	▲	▲▲	▲▲▲
C≠B	*	**	***
B≠A	o	oo	ooo

Fig. 6. Behaviour of systolic and diastolic BP in the same experimental conditions as described in Fig. 4. The two drugs have a similar decreasing action on both SBP and DBP during rest and exercise; Chlorthalidone also has a significant action during recovery.

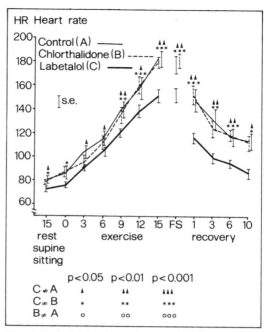

	p<0.05	p<0.01	p<0.001
C≠A	▲	▲▲	▲▲▲
C≠B	*	**	***
B≠A	o	oo	ooo

Fig. 7. Labetalol brings about a significant reduction in heart rate during rest, exercise and recovery, in comparison with the control and with the action of Chlorthalidone.

conditions and randomized using two 3 × 3 Latin squares.

The response to muscular exercise was studied on the cycloergometer with steady loading of 10 watts/min. until the disappearance of the angina or cessation of exercise on account of angina and/or muscular exhaustion, according to the above-described method [4, 5, 6, 7].

During all phases of the experiment the ECG trend was studied using 12 leads, as well as BP (using an aneroid manometer) and the systolic time intervals according to Weissler's method.

The statistical calculation was made by means of Student's test for paired data.

Results

The results may be summarized as follows: Labetalol, to a degree comparable to that of TNG, significantly increased the work load capable of bringing about angina or cessation due to muscular exhaustion (Fig. 8); at the end of the work load period no anginal sensation had been noticed in 3 patients on TNG and 5 on Labetalol.

At the common peak work load for placebo and the two drugs, the degree of deviation below the isoeletric line was clearly reduced after TNG and Labetalol (Fig. 9).

The action mechanism of the two drugs is, in fact, quite different. TNG, confirming the considerable literature on the subject, at the moment of work cessation because of angina or muscular exhaustion has the effect of increased or unvaried double product [10, 11] and a

43

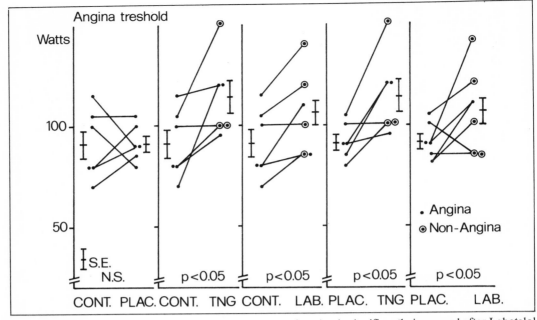

Fig. 8. The work peak wich determines the appearance of angina is significantly increased after Labetalol and TNG as compared to placebo; the exercise was completed without angina by 3 patients on TNG and by 5 on Labetalol.

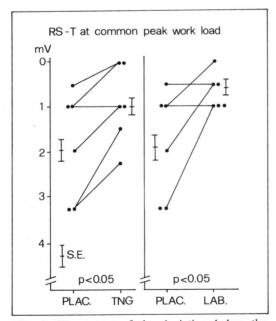

Fig. 9. The extent of the deviation below the isoelectric line at the common peak work load for all three tests (placebo, TNG, Labetalol) is significantly reduced after Labetalol and TNG as compared to placebo.

triple product not very different from that obtained with placebo [10] (Figs. 10 and 11).

The increased double product after TNG treatment means that the anti-ischaemic action of the drug is due to other factors among which the most pre-eminent are considered to be: the reduction in left ventricular volume [12] as a consequence of the reduced venous return flow, the better distribution of blood to the sub-endocardial layers as a result of the reduction in left ventricular telediastolic BP [14] and, perhaps, because of coronary antispastic action.

Labetalol, on the other hand, reduces the double product of HR $\times$ SP and the triple product HR $\times$ SP $\times$ LVET at the moment of angina or of cessation of exercise due to muscular exhaustion.

In the absence of data concerning the behaviour of the contractile state and of ventricular volume after the administration of Labetalol, at the present time at least, it can only be said that the anti-anginal action of Labetalol is largely bound up with the reduced oxygen consumption of the myocardium brought about

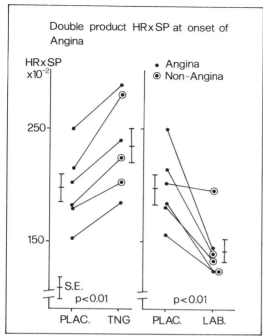

Fig. 10. The product HR ×SP at the onset of angina and the moment of cessation of exercise due to exhaustion increased significantly after TNG and decreased significantly after Labetalol.

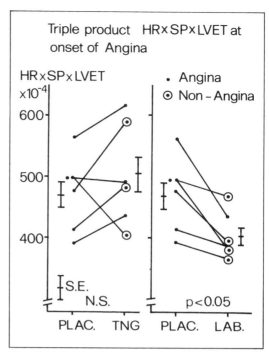

Fig. 11. The product HR ×SP ×LVET at the onset of angina does not differ greatly after TNG as compared to placebo, whereas it is greatly reduced, as compared to placebo, after Labetalol.

by the simultaneous decrease in heart rate and systolic peak.

Remarks

These studies show that the administration of Labetalol can significantly reduce some of the main haemodynamic parameters connected to the oxygen consumption of the myocardium in patients suffering from angina or arterial hypertension.

Particularly in the field of ischaemic heart diseases, the acute, intravenous administration of Labetalol at the 50 mg dose proved capable of significantly reducing the ischaemic modifications and the angina symptoms which appear during effort.

The anti-ischaemic action of Labetalol, at least according to the data currently in our possession, is essentially related to the reduction in postload, as is borne out by the reduction in the double and triple products at the

In conclusion, Labetalol, whether administered acutely or chronically, proved capable moment angina appears, and by the increased exercise required to produce muscular exhaustion.

It remains to be seen whether Labetalol, like Propranolol, has any effect on the contractility of the myocardium and whether, like TNG, it has any effect on the preload, i.e. on the telediastolic volume of the left ventricle.

In has also been proved that Labetalol is able to lower BP after acute and chronic administration, at the same time reducing the double product HR × SP. It is therefore highly probable that the drug can reduce the oxygen consumption of the myocardium, by promoting, through reduction of the postload, the regression of secondary hypertrophic phenomena associated with hypertension.

A particularly favourable effect in anginal hypertensives may also be predicted.

of reducing BP and, at the same time, of decreasing the double product HR $\times$ SP and the triple product HR $\times$ SP $\times$ LVET, haemodynamic parameters related to the oxygen consumption of the myocardium.

However, Labetalol, when administered intravenously proved capable of reducing ischaemic electrocardiographic phenomena and angina symptons in patients suffering from angina, while at the same time reducing the double product of HR $\times$ SP and the triple product of HR $\times$ SP $\times$ LVET.

References

1. Collier J.G., Dawnay N.A.H., Nachev C.H., Robinson B.F.: Clinical investigation of an antagonist at α- and β-adrenoceptors, AH 5158. *Brit. J. Pharmacol*, 44, 286, 1972.
2. Farmer J.B., Kennedy I., Levy G.P., Marshall R.J.: Pharmacology of AH 5158: a drug which blocks both α- and β-adrenoceptors. *Brit. J. Pharmacol.*, 45, 660, 1972.
3. Cherchi A., Raffo M., Sau F., Seguro C., Pirisi R.: Azione del labetalolo sulla frequenza cardiaca, sulla pressione arteriosa e sui tempi sistolici a riposo e sotto sforzo in soggetti ipertesi. *Boll. Soc. Ital. Cardiol.*, 23, 158, 1978.
4. Cherchi A., Nissardi G.P., Raffo M., Maxia L.: Electrocardiogramme et metabolisme au cours de l'effort chez les normaux et les cardiaques. Un test calibré pour l'évaluation de l'insuffisance coronaire. *Memorias IV Congreso Mondial de Cardiologia*, II, 224, Mexico, 1962.
5. Lenti G., Cherchi A., Raffo M., Porrazzo G.: Una prova da sforzo tarata con carichi progressivamente crescenti per la diagnosi elettrocardiografica dell'insufficienza coronarica. *Minerva Med*, 57, 418, 1966.
6. Weissler A.M., Harris W.S., Schoenfeld C.D.: Bedside techniques for the evaluation of ventricular function in man. *Amer. J. Cardiol.*, 23, 577, 1969.
7. Cherchi A., Montaldo P.L., Sau F.: Sulle variazioni degli intervalli sistolici nel corso dell'esercizio muscolare in rapporto all'età e al sesso. *Boll. Soc. Ital. Cardiol.*, 23, 110, 1978.
8. Raffo M., Cherchi A., Sau F., Pirisi R., Seguro C., Pisano M.R.: Effetto del labetalolo e del clortalidone sulla tolleranza allo sforzo in soggetti ipertesi. *Boll. Soc. Ital. Cardiol.* 24, 657, 1979.
9. Cherchi A., Fonzo R., Lai C., Mercuro G.: Influenza del labetalolo sul test di tolleranza allo sforzo in pazienti affetti da angina pectoris. *Boll. Soc. Ital. Cardiol.*, 23, 281, 1978.
10. Goldstein R.E.: Clinical and circulatory effects of isosorbite dinitrate. Comparison with nitroglycerin. *Circulation*, 43, 629, 1971.
11. Cherchi A., Fonzo R., Bina M.: Influenza sul test di tolleranza allo sforzo della TNG, del propranololo, dell'amiodarone e del placebo nell'angina pectoris. *Boll. Soc. Ital. Cardiol.*, 19, 1491, 1974.
12. Williams J.F. Jr., Glick G., Braunwald E.: Studies on cardiac dimensions in intact unanesthetized man. V. Effects of nitroglycerin. *Circulation*, 32, 767, 1965.
13. Fonzo R., Cherchi A., Lai C., Cioglia G., Mercuro G., Bina P.: Effetto della trinitroglicerina sulle dimensioni ecocardiografiche del ventricolo sinistro nella cardiopatia ischemica: confronto con placebo. *Boll. Soc. Ital. Cardiol.*, 24, 383, 1979.
14. Kjekshus J.K.: Mechanism for flow distribution in normal and ischemic myocardium during increased ventricular preload in the dog. *Circ. Res.*, 33, 489, 1973.

Hypertension, recent advances and research
edited by M. Condorelli, A. Zanchetti
Cortina International, Verona 1982

Adrenoceptor blockade in the treatment of hypertension: haemodynamic implications

G. KOCH

Department of Clinical Physiology, Central Hospital, Karlskrona, Sweden, and Department of Physiology, Free University of Berlin, West Berlin.

Key words. Adrenoceptor Blockade; Early Hypertension; Established Hypertension; Late Hypertension; Haemodynamic Pattern; Labetalol; Beta-receptor Blockade; Alpha-adrenoceptor Blockade; Combined Alpha-beta-blockade; Systemic Vascular Resistances, Left Ventricular Filling Pressure; Cardio-selective Beta-receptor Antagonists; Non-selective Beta-receptor Antagonists; Long-term Therapy; Cardiovascular Dynamics.

Summary. The haemodynamic pattern in hypertension varies according to the age of the subject and the stage of the hypertensive disorder. In the early stage, both cardiac output and systemic vascular resistance tend to be elevated. Advanced stages are characterized by a hypokinetic type of circulation with subnormal cardiac output and considerably increased systemic vascular resistance.

Both cardioselective and non-selective beta-receptor antagonists lower cardiac output and tend to raise systemic vascular resistance. Even left ventricular filling pressure tends to be higher. While these effects are most distinct in the acute experiment, cardiac output always remains depressed and systemic vascular resistance often remains at a higher level as compared with pre-treatment values, even during long-term therapy. Intrinsic sympathetic activity may attenuate, but does not abolish these effects. The anti-hypertensive action of beta-receptor blockers appears to be mainly due to the reduction in cardiac output.

Post-synaptic alpha (alpha-1) receptor blockers reduce blood pressure by a substantial decrease in systemic vascular resistance and tend to raise stroke volume and cardiac output, in particular during exercise. Left ventricular filling pressure tends towards lower levels. Heart rate increases only moderately.

Combined alpha-beta-blockade lowers blood pressure predominantly by alpha-receptor-mediated reduction of systemic vascular resistance both when induced acutely and during long-term administration. Due to its beta-receptor blocking component the increase in cardiac output is abolished: cardiac output is mainly maintained at pre-treatment levels as is left ventricular filling pressure.

Since a well balanced blockade of both alpha- and beta-receptors counteracts the haemodynamic changes occurring in the course of hypertension and tends to restore cardiovascular dynamics to normal, combined alpha-beta-receptor blockade appears to be one of the most logical and rational therapeutical approaches to hypertension.

Drug therapy of systemic arterial hypertension is still mainly based on trial and error, the only criterion of efficacy, in general, being the degree of blood-pressure reduction achivied. It is evident that lowering of blood presure to preferably normal levels must remain the prime concern of physicians; it is, however, also obvious that, ideally, anti-hypertensive treatment should not only aim at lowering systemic blood pressure, but should achieve this by reversing the pathophysiological changes induced by the disease process. That implies, of course, that, in choosing an anti-hypertensive agent, factors such as age of the subject and stage of the disease, and the pharmacological profile of the drug have to be taken into account. Since hypertension is primarily a circulatory disorder prompting above all cardiovascular changes and often morbid cardiovascular events, haemodynamic aspects must reasonably play a cardinal rôle in all therapeutical considerations.

The purpose of this paper is to briefly review the haemodynamic consequences of adrenoceptor blockade in hypertensive patients; since different haemodynamic patterns, however, are seen in the course of hypertension a short review of its natural history in terms of haemodynamics is given as well.

The haemodynamic pattern of hypertension

Irrespective of which causative mechanisms may eventually be involved in the multifactorial disorder called essential hypertension, it is axiomatic that such mechanisms would have to influence blood pressure through changes in cardiac output or in systemic vascular resistance, or in both of these variables. During the last 15 years it has become evident that their mutual importance in generating high blood pressure differs depending upon the age of the subject and the stage of the hypertensive disorder [5, 15, 17, 18].

Early essential hypertension

In younger subjects (18 to 29 years) with mild essential hypertension, cardiac output at rest is usually higher than in normotensive age-matched controls; stroke volume is usually normal; heart rate is increased. Total systemic vascular resistance, however, is within normal limits.

This increased cardiac output in early essential hypertension is often referred to as a "hyperkinetic" circulation. However, the observation that oxygen uptake is also increased indicates that the rise cardiac output corresponds to an increase in metabolic rate. The cause of this abnormality is unknown; it might be related to increased sympathetic activity which has been shown to exist in hypertensives at this stage compared with age-matched controls [11,12] (Fig. 1). During exercise a different haemodynamic pattern is seen: cardiac output is no longer high, but rather subnormal. During maximal exercise it is significantly lower than in age-matched controls when related to oxygen uptake. Surprisingly enough, stroke volume is lower than in agematched controls. This is partly compensated for by an increased heart rate, but the compensation falls short during strenuous exercise. Furthermore, total systemic resistance during exercise does not fall to the levels seen in normotensive controls.

Thus, already in subjects with mild WHO stage I essential hypertension, some kind of left ventricular function disturbance as well as alterations in vascular resistance are present; they are reflected in a subnormal stroke volume during exercise an by a lowe degree of exercise-induced vasodilation [15].

Established hypertension

In subjects older than 30 years with mild-to-moderate established hypertension (WHO stages I and II), cardiac output at rest is usually normal; total systemic resistance is increased. During exercise cardiac output becomes subnormal, even at lower levels of activity, and is associated with a subnormal strike volume and high heart rate. The arteriovenous oxygen difference is increased. Total systemic resistance is significantly raised both at rest and during exercise.

Late and severe hypertension

Finally, in subjects with marked blood pressure elevation and in particular in patients showing target organ damage (WHO stage III) stroke volume is small and cardiac output is low, both at rest and during exercise. Systemic resistance is grossly elevated. With progressing left ventricular function disturbance, in addition, left ventricular filling pressures gradually increase.

Changes in the haemodynamic pattern

The findings in cross-sectional studies of specific haemodynamic patterns at different

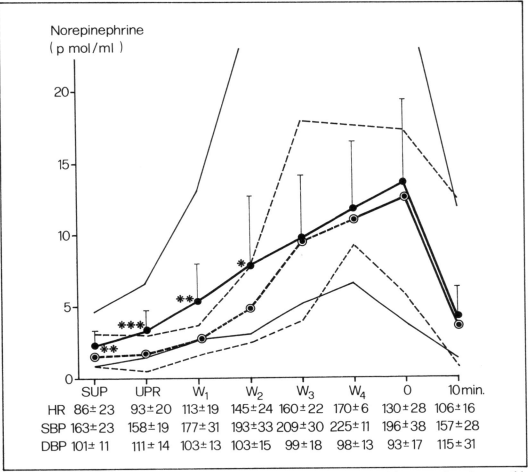

Fig. 1. Plasma norepinephrine in a group of normotensive young adults (n = 16, means: ◉ and range: thin broken line) and a group of age-matched WHO stage I hypertensives (n = 14, means; ●, standard deviations and range: solid line) at rest, supine and upright, and during ergometer exercise sitting at different work loads (W_1: 50, W_2: 100, W_3: 150, W_4: 200 Watt) and after exercise again in the supine position. Heart rates (HR, beats/min), systolic (SBP, mmHg) and diastolic (DBP, mmHg) blood pressures are given for the group of hypertensives only. Note the significantly higher plasma norepinephrine levels in the hypertensives during resting conditions and during light exercise, but not during heavy exercise (*: $p < 0.05$, **: $p < 0.01$, ***: $p < 0.001$).

ages and disease stages strongly suggest a gradual change taking place in long-standing hypertension from the early, so-called hyperkinetic pattern to the hypokinetic high resistance pattern. However, only recent longitudinal studies have definitely established that these haemodynamic alterations actually do occur in the course of hypertension [17, 18]. Two groups of patients with mild hypertension, under 40 years of age when initially seen, were re-examined after a 10-year period without treatment. Although only small changes in blood pressure had occurred during rest, the haemodynamic pattern itself had changed. Cardiac output had decreased and total peripheral resistance had increased more than would have been expected from aging alone. The decrease in cardiac output was mainly due to a decrease in stroke volume.

During exercise, corresponding blood pressures were higher after the 10-year interval, in particular during the highest work load. Cardiac output during exercise was significantly lower than 10 years earlier, mainly due to a decrease in stroke volume, while peripheral resistance was higher.

Haemodynamics following adrenoceptor blockade

Interpretation of the haemodynamic effects of drugs that competitively antagonize adrenoceptors in the heart and the vascular system is compounded by a number of difficulties. These include: the effects on isolated heart muscle may be quite different from the effects of the compounds on the intact heart; interference with the pumping activity of the heart and/or vascular regulation has immediate reflex effects throughout the circulation aimed at counteracting these changes; the haemodynamic effects of sympatholytic drugs are in direct proportion to the amount of adrenergic drive reigning at the time. Furthermore, the haemodynamic effect in intact man may be misleading if applied to interpretation of the effects in pathological circulatory conditions. These problems of analysis and interpretation are illustrated by the finding that, in the normal intact heart under minimal sympathetic stimulation, beta-receptor antagonists have relatively little haemodynamic activity; yet in the heart under intense sympathetic drive, such as during exercise or in the heart partially depleted of sympathetic neurotransmitters, as in heart failure, these drugs exert profound effects.

It is against such a background and with all these limitations in mind, that the haemodynamic activity of any adrenoceptor blocking drug must be examined and interpreted. However, although haemodynamic effects might be difficult to dissect into their component sources, they will nevertheless allow important conclusions concerning the overall cardiovascular action of adrenoceptor-blockade. At worst, they will allow the prescription to be formulated for any given pathophysiological state. Since exercise induces a fairly reproducible state of adrenergic activity, the study of the haemodynamic response to exercise has become an essential part of all reliable analyses of the cardiovascular effects of adrenergic antagonists.

Haemodynamic effects of beta-receptor blockade

The basic haemodynamic effects of beta-adrenoceptor blockade have been established using the first beta-receptor antagonist applied on a wide scale, propranolol [6, 28]. The acute i.v. or oral administration of a beta-blocker such as propranolol leads to a decrease in heart rate and cardiac output and a widening of the arteriovenous oxygen difference compensating for the fall in cardiac output and ensuring unchanged oxygen transport capacity. As a response to the reduction of cardiac output the total systemic vascular resistance is raised and prevents systemic blood pressure from being substantially lowered. In the intact heart, left ventricular filling pressures and stroke volume are mainly unchanged or show a tendency towards slightly higher levels; the haemodynamic changes become in general more pronounced during exercise. However, when treatment is prolonged for months or years, the systemic vascular resistance shows some regression towards pre-treatment levels; due to this readjustment blood pressure falls in the so-called "responders". In the "non-responders" vascular resistance remains at the initial level [7].

During the last 15 years a large number of beta-receptor blockers has been introduced in the therapy of hypertension. They may be divided into 4 main groups (Table I): non-cardioselective and cardioselective, and, within each group, compounds with or without intrinsic sympathetic activity (ISA). If the so-called membrane-stabilizing (or quinidine-like) effect is taken into account, further subgroups emerge.

Basically, all these compounds show a haemodynamic profile very similar to that of propranolol. Thus, in the acute experiment, cardiac output is decreased and systemic vascular resistance rises; a distinct hypotensive effect is usually lacking and becomes evident

Table I. *Classification of beta-adrenoceptor blocking drugs.*

Non-selective	Partial agonist effect (ISA)	Membrane-stabilizing effect
1. Non-selective $(\beta_1 + \beta_2)$ block		
Group 1 Oxprenolol	+	+
Alprenolol	+	+
Group 2 Propranolol	−	+
Penbutolol	−	+
Group 3 Pindolol	+	−
Group 4 Sotalol	−	−
Timolol	−	−
Nadolol	−	−
2. Cardioselective (β_1) block		
Group 1 Acebutolol	+	+
Group 3 Practolol	+	−
Group 4 Atenolol	−	−
Metoprolol	−	−
3. Non-selective block + alpha-block		
Group 2 Labetalol	−	+
4. Cardioselective block + alpha-block		
No example yet available		

only during prolonged treatment. For some of these drugs, in particular pindolol, it has been claimed that the haemodynamic profile during long-term treatment differs substantially from that seen with propranolol. Atterhög [1] has actually found cardiac output to be restored to, and systemic vascular resistance lowered below, pre-treatment values after 16 months of treatment with pindolol. The recent studies of Lund-Johansen [20] are of particular interest in this context since he studied the haemodynamic effects of quite a number of different beta-blockers using strictly identical methods (intravascular blood pressure measurement, dye-dilution determination of cardiac output) and age-matched patients with slight stage 1-2 essential hypertension. Mean duration of treatment was one year; the doses used were equipotential (Fig. 2). These studies clearly demonstrate that basically, the changes induced are similar to those seen with propranolol. Heart rate and cardiac output were reduced between 11 and 30% at rest and during exercise (Fig. 3); however, vascular resistance did not change uniformly (Fig. 4); thus, in the timolol group systemic vascular resistance re-

mained significantly elevated, whereas this parameter was reversed to pre-treatment levels during treatment with atenolol, penbutolol and, in particular, pindolol. However, with no beta-receptor antagonist did the vascular resistance significantly fall below pre-treatment values. Surprisingly enough, the 4 beta-blockers that showed the most favourable effect on vascular resistance at rest, supine and during exercise in this series belonged to totally different groups; two non-selective blockers with ISA: alprenolol and pindolol; one non-selective without ISA: penbutolol and one cardioselective without ISA: atenolol. Prolongation of treatment up to five years did not induce any further change as demonstrated for atenolol [19].

Concerning pressures in the pulmonary circulation and, in particular, left ventricular filling pressures, information is very scanty. In the studies available, a tendency towards higher pressures has been shown. This was the case even in a group of WHO stage 1-2 hypertensives that were restudied after one year of treatment with the non-selective blocker oxprenolol in combination with the vasodilator hydralazine [9]. Surprisingly enough the overall

51

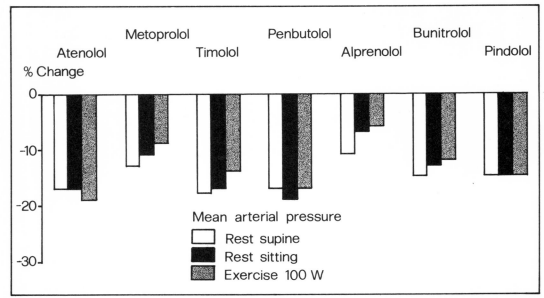

Fig. 2. Effect of different beta-receptor antagonists on systemic mean blood pressure at rest and during exercise in different groups of age-matched hypertensives, WHO stage I. Doses were equipotential and treatment lasted for one year. According to data presented by Lund-Johansen[20], by permission of the author.

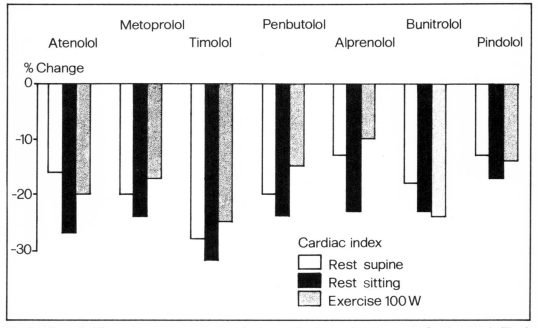

Fig. 3. Effect of different beta-receptor antagonists on cardiac index. Same groups of patients as in Fig. 2. According to data presented by Lund-Johansen[20], by permission of the author.

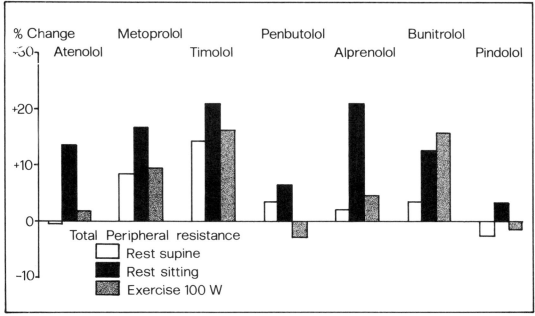

Fig. 4. Effect of different beta-receptor antagonists on total systemic resistance. Same groups of patients as in Figs. 2 and 3. The data were recalculated from the data given in Figs. 2 and 3 with the permission of the author. Note that the increase in total peripheral resistance was statistically significant only after metoprolol at rest sitting ($p < 0.04$), after timolol during all conditions (supine: $p < 0.05$, sitting: $p < 0.01$, exercise: $p < 0.01$), and after alprenolol and bunitrolol again during sitting conditions ($p < 0.05$).

haemodynamic pattern observed with this combination did not differ substantially from that seen with a pure beta-receptor blocker.

This might, however, be due to the rather high dose of oxprenolol (480 mg daily) used in this series.

However, the increases in pulmonary and left ventricular filling pressures seen with beta-blockade seldom reach levels of clinical significance except in patients exhibiting distinct left ventricular function disturbance or dyskinesia.

Haemodynamic effects of alpha-adrenoceptor blockade

Since constriction of the peripheral resistance vessels is predominantly mediated through alpha-adrenoceptors, alpha-receptor blockade would appear to be the most logical therapeutical approach. Agents with alpha-blocking or other vasodilator properties, such as phento-

lamine, hydralazine and minoxidil, have regularly been shown to reduce systemic vascular resistance and thereby blood pressure in man [29]. However, the pressure decrease usually activates the homeostatic baroreceptor mechanism, thus causing an increase in heart rate and cardiac output. This secondary effect has in the past limited the usefulness of vasodilators or alpha-blockers as antihypertensive agents.

During recent years prazosin has met with increasing interest; the discussion of the haemodynamic effects of alpha-blockade will be mainly restricted to this compound. Early studies suggested that prazosin was a peripheral vasodilator, this effect being due to both alpha-adrenoceptor blockade and direct smooth muscle relaxation. Currently, however, on the basis of in-vitro studies, prazosin is believed to be a selective post-synaptic alpha-adrenoceptor blocking agent [4].

Surprisingly, there are hardly any haemodynamic studies of the acute effect of prazosin in hypertensive patients using reliable methods including exercise. It appears, however, at least during resting conditions, that there is an immediate fall in blood pressure entirely due to a reduction in systemic vascular resistance [21]. Heart rate and cardiac output increase, if at all, only insignificantly. Judging from studies in patients with left ventricular failure, left ventricular filling pressures are reduced. There appears to be but one study concerning long-term haemodynamic adaptation to prazosin monotherapy in hypertensives. After one year's treatment, CO during exercise was found to be significantly increased due to larger stroke volume, the substantial reduction in systemic vascular resistance being preserved [16].

A number of studies has demonstrated the drastic reduction in preload and afterload, and increase in stroke volume and cardiac output of prazosin in left ventricular failure [2, 3]. As with other vasodilators the effect appears the more pronounced, the higher the left ventricular pressure.

The absence of significant increases in heart rate following prazosin, as should be expected to occur due to the baroreflex mechanism, is surprising; it has been attributed to the drug's property of only blocking post-synaptic alpha-receptors leaving the negative feedback inhibition of increased noradrenal release via pre-synaptic alpha-receptors intact. The non-selective (pre- and post-synaptic) alpha-receptor blocker phentolamine does not possess these properties and actually leads to a significant increase in heart rate and cardiac output.

Haemodynamic effects of combined alpha-beta-blockade

Not only from a theoretical but also from a practical point of view, the combination of a vasodilator or alpha-receptor blocking agent with a beta-adrenoceptor antagonist appears attractive and logical. First, the anti-hypertensive effect of the vasodilator is increased by additional beta-receptor blockade; second, due to the alpha-receptor blocking component, blood pressure can be expected to be lowered predominantly by a reduction in systemic vascular resistance while a possible reflex increase in cardiac output would be attenuated or prevented by the beta-blocking component. Furthermore, activation of the renin-angiotensin system regularly seen after vasodilation and/or alpha-receptor blockade would be suppressed; the additional reduction in blood pressure achieved by adding a beta-receptor antagonist to a vasodilator drug regimen has actually been claimed to be dependent on a renin-suppressing action of the beta-receptor antagonist in this situation [23].

Unfortunately, only one reliable haemodynamic study of the combined effects of prazosin plus beta-blocker appears available [18]. Prazosin, 4 mg daily, in combination with the cardioselective beta-receptor antagonist tolalomol, 200 mg daily, decreased blood pressure more efficiently than prazosin, 4 mg daily, alone. As expected, after one year's combination treatment, systemic vascular resistance was found to be diminished, in particular during exercise but cardiac output also tended to be lower. A similar haemodynamic pattern was demonstrated in 3 patients after a 3-month treatment with alprenolol in combination with dihydralazine [24], while the aforementioned study of the combined effects of oxprenolol (450 mg daily) and hydralazine (150 mg daily) failed to demonstrate a significant reduction in systemic vascular resistance [9]. Apparently, the haemodynamic pattern obtained depends to a large degree on the effective dose relationship between vasodilator or alpha-blocker and beta-receptor antagonist.

Labetalol constitutes a unique compound in this context since it combines in the same molecule an alpha-adrenoceptor blocking action, predominantly at the post-synaptic site, with beta-adrenoceptor blocking properties. The beta-receptor antagonist component is non-cardioselective and lacks intrinsic sympathetic activity, but has membrane-stabilizing properties (Table I). In a series of haemodynamic studies [10, 11, 12] we could demonstrate that Labetalol not only produces haemodynamic effects in accordance with what could be anticipated from its pharmacological profile but

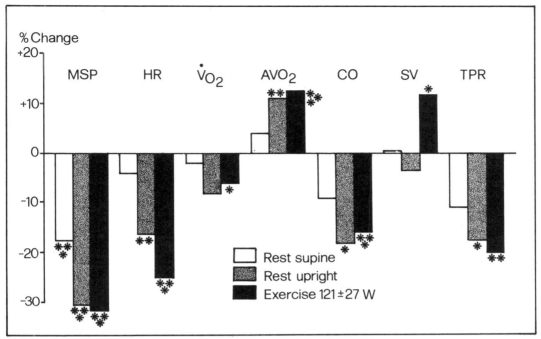

Fig. 5. Percentage changes from pre-treatment values of some haemodynamic variables at rest and during exercise, after intravenous administration of Labetalol 50 mg[10]; MSP: mean systemic pressure, HR: heart rate, VO_2: oxygen uptake, AVO_2; arterio-mixed venous oxygen difference, CO: cardiac output, SV: stroke volume, TPR: total peripheral resistances. *: $p < 0.05$, **: $p < 0.01$, ***: $p < 0.001$.

that the balance between alpha- and beta-receptor blocking activity is very appropriate in the majority of cases.

The acute administration of Labetalol, 50 mg intravenously, induced in our series a significant fall in systemic blood pressure under all conditions; at rest, supine and upright and during steady-state bicycle ergometer exercise, it was due to a reduction in both systemic vascular resistance and cardiac output, in particular during exercise (Fig. 5). The decrease in cardiac output was entirely due to a reduction in heart rate. The arterio-mixed venous oxygen difference changed inversely with the alterations in cardiac output. After a long-term, i.e. 20-month, period of oral treatment, average dose 900 mg daily, the reduction in blood pressure was maintained, but was now entirely due to a decrease in systemic vascular resistance, while cardiac output was brought back to pre-treatment levels (Fig. 6). The rise in cardiac output was due to an increase in stroke volume which entirely counterbalanced the fall in heart rate. This effect was particularly important in the upright position. After long-term oral treatment, the stroke volume in the upright position was actually of the same order as the supine stroke volume prior to treatment. This explains why postural hypotension, which frequently occurred after the acute administration of Labetalol, had practically disappeared during the course of oral treatment. It is noteworthy that intrapulmonary pressures, including left ventricular filling pressures, and left ventricular performance characteristics in terms of stroke volume/filling pressure ratio were not significantly altered [11]; this clearly suggests that the negative inotropic effect of the beta-blocking component is counterbalanced by the concomitant alpha-blockade.

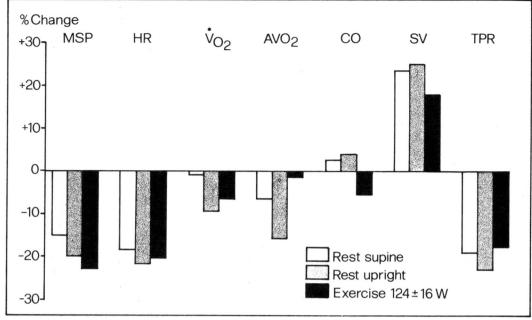

Fig. 6. Percentage changes from pre-treatment values of some haemodynamic variables at rest and during exercise, after 20 months' oral treatment with Labetalol, average daily dose 900 mg.[11] Abbreviations and symbols as in Fig. 5.

Conclusions

It is apparent from this overview that all anti-hypertensive regimens using one or another type of adrenergic receptor blockade generally lead to a reduction in systemic blood pressure; however, the mechanism by which this is achieved varies quite substantially. There is a wide range from significant depression of cardiac output and rise in systemic vascular resistance to increase in cardiac output and reduction in vascular resistance (Table II).

Although an anti-hypertensive regimen that lowers blood pressure and normalizes the haemodynamic alterations following the hypertensive disorder clearly appears more logical and attractive, there is at present no proof that treatment with such a "physiological" regimen indeed carries a better prognosis regarding life expectancy and cardiovascular events.

Table II. *Changes in some haemodynamic variables and in plasma renin activity usually occurring during treatment with beta-receptor antagonists, alpha-1-receptor antagonist and alpha-beta-adrenoceptor blockers.*

	Beta-receptor blockade	Alpha-receptor blockade (prazosin)	Alpha-beta-receptor blockade
Heart rate	decreased	increased or unchanged	decreased or unchanged
Cardiac output	decreased	increased or unchanged	unchanged
Stroke volume	unchanged or increased	increased or unchanged	increased or unchanged
Systemic vascular resistance	increased or unchanged	decreased	decreased
Arterio-venous oxygen differ.	increased	decreased or unchanged	unchanged or increased
Left ventricular filling pres.	increased	decreased	unchanged
Plasma Renin Activity (PRA)	decreased	increased or unchanged	decreased

While it appears doubtful that studies aimed at establishing such evidence for various reasons will or can ever be undertaken, studies of the effect of treatment on organ perfusion give indirect evidence that a regimen which does not significantly lower cardiac output may be advantageous. Though information on the effects of different antihypertensive principles on the distribution of cardiac output is scanty, the data available clearly suggest that, generally, perfusion in most vital vascular beds closely follows the changes in the central circulation and, in particular, cardiac output.

Thus, renal blood flow has been shown to be reduced after the acute administration of Labetalol and metoprolol [11] in proportion to the changes in cardiac output, i.e. by 10 and 15 per cent respectively. Similar reductions in glomerular filtration rates to those observed after the acute administration of Labetalol and metoprolol have been reported to subsist during long-term treatment with propranolol [8]. Liver blood flow has been found to fall more than would be expected from the reduction in systemic arterial pressure again during prolonged beta-adrenoceptor blockade with propranolol [26, 27] thus indicating an increase in hepatic vascular resistance. Significant reductions in liver perfusion could have implications for the metabolism of some of the adrenoceptor antagonists themselves. Studies of the response of skeletal muscle blood flow to chronic beta-receptor blockade [26, 27] show that similar reductions in perfusion occur even in the vascular bed of the working muscle. Furthermore, a whole series of clinical observations indicates that the incidence of leg symptoms attributable to reduced muscle flow is higher with beta-receptor blockers inducing significant reductions in cardiac output than with agents having but minor effects on cardiac output. This supports the view that changes in regional perfusion correspond to the changes in central haemodynamics. There is possibly one exception to this rule: judging from the results obtained in primates, it appears that cerebral blood flow is relatively less reduced than blood flow in other vascular beds [22].

References

1. Atterhög, J.H., Dunér, H.B.: Haemodynamic effects of pindolol in hypertensive patients. *Acta Med. Scand.* Suppl. 606, 55, 1977.

2. Awan, N.A., Miller, R.R., De Maria, A.N., Maxwell, K.S., Neumann, A., Mason, D.: Efficacy of ambulatory systemic vasodilator therapy with oral prazosin in chronic refractory heart failure. *Circulation* 56, 346, 1977.

3. Awan, N.A., Miller, R.R., Mason, D.T.: Comparison of effects of nitroprusside and prazosin on left ventricular function and the peripheral circulation in chronic refractory congestive heart failure. *Circulation* 57, 152, 1978.

4. Cambridge, D., Davey, M.J., Nassingham, R.: Prazosin, a selective antagonist of postsynaptic α-adrenoceptors. *Brit. J. Pharmacol.* 59, 514, 1977.

5. Freis, E.D.: Hemodynamics in hypertension. *Physiol. Rev.* 40, 27, 1960.

6. Furberg, C., von Schmalensee, G.: Beta-adrenergic blockade and central circulation during exercise in sitting position in healthy subjects. *Acta Physiol. Scand.* 73, 435, 1968.

7. Hansson, L.: Beta-adrenergic blockade in essential hypertension. Effects of propranolol on hemodynamic parameters and plasma renin activity. *Acta Med. Scand.* Suppl. 550, 49, 1973.

8. Ibsen, H., Sederberg-Olsen, P.: Changes in glomerular filtration rate during long-term treatment with propranolol in patients with arterial hypertension. *Clin. Sci. Mol. Med.* 44, 129, 1973.

9. Koch, G.: Hemodynamic adaptation at rest and during exercise to long-term antihypertensive treatment with combination of beta-receptor blocking and vasodilator agent. *Brit Heart J.*, 38, 1240, 1976.

10. Koch, G.: Acute hemodynamic effects of an alpha- and beta-receptor blocking agent (AH 5158) on the systemic and pulmonary circulation at rest and during exercise in hypertensive patients. *Amer. Heart J.*, 93, 585, 1977.

11. Koch, G.: Haemodynamic adaptation at rest and during exercise to long-term antihypertensive treatment with combined alpha- and beta-adrenoreceptor blockade by labetalol. *Brit. Heart J.* 41, 192, 1979.

12. Koch, G.: Cardiovascular dynamics after acute and long-term alpha- and beta-adrenoceptor blockade at rest, supine and standing and during exercise. *Brit. J. Clin. Pharmacol.* 8, 101 s, 1979.

13. Koch, G.: Effects of cardioselective beta-receptor blockade and of combined alpha-beta-receptor blockade on renal dynamics and on adrenergic activity. Abstracts, *6th Scientific Meeting of the International Society of Hypertension*, Goteborg, p. 145, 1979.

14. Koch, G.: Exercise adreno-sympathetic activity in essential hypertension. *Pflügers Archiv (Eur. J. Physiol.)* 379, R 35, 1979.

15. Lund-Johansen, P.: Hemodynamics in early essential hypertension. *Acta Med. Scand.* Suppl. 428, 1, 1967

16. Lund-Johansen, P.: Haemodynamic changes at rest

and during exercise in long-term prazosin therapy of essential hypertension. In Cotton. D.W.K. (Ed.) *Prazosin: Evaluation of a new antihypertensive agent.* Amsterdam Excerpta Medica, pp. 45-53, 1974.

17. Lund-Johansen, P.: Central hemodynamics in essential hypertension. *Acta Med. Scand.* Suppl. 606, 35, 1977.

18. Lund-Johansen, P.: Hemodynamic long-term effects of prazosin plus tolamolol in essential hypertension. *Brit J. Clin. Pharmacol.* 4, 141-145, 1977.

19. Lund-Johansen, P.: Hemodynamic consequences of long-term beta-blocker therapy: a 5-year follow-up study of atenolol. *J. Cardiovasc. Pharmacol.* 1; 487, 1979.

20. Lund-Johansen, P.: The effect of beta-blocker therapy on chronic hemodynamics. *Primary Cardiology* Suppl. 1, 20, 1980.

21. Mancia, G., Ferran, A., Gregorini, L., Ferrari, M.C., Bianchini, C., Terzoli, Leonetti, G. and Zanchetti, A.: Regulation of the circulation during antihypertensive treatment with prazosin. In: Rawlins M.D., Geyer G., Bleifeld. M., (Eds) *Proceedings of the European Prazosin Symposium* 1979, Amsterdam, Excerpta Medica 1979, p 15.

22. Nies, A.S., Evans, G.H., Shand, D.G.: Regional hemodynamic effects of beta-adrenergic blockade with propranolol in the unanesthetized primate. *Amer. Heart J.*, 85, 97, 1973.

23. Pettinger, W.A., Mitchell, M.C.: Renin release, savalasin and vasodilator beta-blocker drug interaction in man. *New Engl. J. Med.*, 292, 1214, 1975.

24. Sannerstedt, R.: Selection of hypertensive patients for treatment with beta-blockers alone or in combination. In: W. Schweitzer. (Ed.) *Beta-blockers: Present status and future prospects.* Basel, Hans Huber, 1975.

25. Sivertsson, R.: Peripheral haemodynamics in essential hypertension. *Acta Med. Scand.* Suppl 606, 43, 1977.

26. Trap-Jensen, J., Clausen, J.P., Noer, I., Mogensen, A., Christensen, M. J., Krogsgaard, A.R., Larsen, O.A.: Regional hemodynamic changes during exercise in essential hypertension before and after prolonged beta-receptor blockade. *Scand J. Clin. Lab. Invest.* 35, Suppl. 143, 60, 1975.

27. Trap-Jensen, J. Clausen, J.P., Noer, I., Larsen, O.A., Krogsgaard, A.R., Christensen, N.J.: The effects of beta-adrenoceptor blockers on cardiac output, liver blood flow and skeletal muscle blood flow in hypertensive patients. *Acta Physiol. Scand.* 98, Suppl. 440, 30, 1976.

28. Ulrych, M., Frohlich, E.D., Dustan, M.P., Page, I.H.: Immediate hemodynamic effects of beta-adrenergic blockade with propranolol in normotensive and hypertensive man. *Circulation* 37, 411, 1968.

29. Zacest, R.: The clinical pharmacology of hypotensive vasodilator drugs. *Med. J. Aust.*, Suppl. 1, 4, 1975.

Hypertension, recent advances and research
edited by M. Condorelli, A. Zanchetti
Cortina International, Verona 1982

Clinical and echocardiographic studies in the acute and chronic treatment of hypertension

F. PLASTINA, F. CURIA, N. VENNERI, M. CHIATTO
Department of Cardiology, Cosenza Civic Hospital

Key words. Hypertension; Echocardiography; Labetalol; Propranolol; Left Ventricular Performance; Left Ventricular Dimensions; Acute Treatment; Chronic Treatment; Diastolic Diameter; Systolic Diameter; Percentage of Systolic Contaction.

Summary.   Ten patients were administered an acute i.v. dose of Labetalol (fast bolus of 50 mg in 1 min.). BP values in the supine position are noticeably reduced; after 30 min. there was seen to be a decrease in systolic and diastolic values of 32.5 and 11 mmHg respectively.
HR and the LV performance and dimensions parameters, recorded by M-mode echocardiography before treatment and after 10, 20, and 30 min., remained virtually unchanged as compared to basal values.
A clinical and echocardiographic study was carried out following the chronic administration of Labetalol. The 15 patients with uncomplicated essential hypertension were given a therapeutically efficacious dose of Labetalol (varying between 300 and 900 mg/day). The patients were examined in basal conditions and after 20 and 60 days of treatment. At the end of the study, supine BP values showed a reduction of 19 mmHg (systolic) and 18 mmHg (diastolic). LV performance and dimensions did not change substantially, according to the echocardiographic recordings; HR underwent a slight but not significant decrease (-8.3 after 60 days). In 8 of the above group of patients, Labetalol was replaced by Propranolol in adequate doses to achieve the same therapeutic effect and a clinical echocardiographic check was made after 20 and 60 days. In comparison with Labetalol, Propranolol brings about a more marked slowing of HR (-18.5 in comparison with the values obtained with Labetalol), an increase in DSD and an increase (not so marked) in SSD. Vcf diminishes, but not in a statistically significant way. Nevertheless, the substantial non-variation of S% suggests that the changes found can be largely attributed to the marked decrease in HR after treatment with Propranolol.

Introduction

The definition of the echocardiographic image of the endocardium and of the septum and the posterior wall has made possible numerous observations of the morphology and function of the left ventricle.

The ultrasonic beam, following an antero-posterior route, whilst exploring a limited part of the left ventricle (using M-mode), permits the determination of the telediastolic and telesystolic dimensions, morphology, thickness and movement of the septum and the posterior wall [1].

The good correlation between the internal echocardiographic dimensions and the angiocardiographic volumes inspired research aimed at obtaining information about more complex parameters (ventricular volume, cardiac output, ejection fraction, ventricular mass, etc.) from the simple linear dimensions [2, 3, 4, 5].

The geometric hypothesis on which the assumption is based (i.e. that the echocardiographic axis corresponds to a short angiocardiographic axis) cannot be applicable in the case of dilated hearts or hearts with hypokinesis of the walls. Later experience therefore made clear that important errors of calculation are the result of the application in cardiac pathology of the proposed formulae, both the initial formulae based on raising the internal echocardiographic dimensions to the cubic power and the later, more accurate formulae based on regression equations [6]. The linear determination of the ventricular dimensions is true echocardiographic measurement and a useful point of reference, without further elaborations which add to or multiply the methodological errors [7].

Thanks to its repeatability, innocuousness and low cost, ultrasound cardiography is currently a singular and original way of providing programmed monitoring of ventricular function and dimensions in cardiopathic patients and of checking the effects of drugs on specific parameters. In this case, the method is rendered valid by the fact that each patient is his own control.

Over the last few years, many studies using ultrasound cardiography have demonstrated the modification of certain ventricular functions and dimensions after the administration of cardio- and vaso-active drugs [8, 9, 10, 11, 12, 13, 23]. The usefulness of echocardiography for assessing left ventricular morphology and function in a group of slight and moderate hypertensives has been proved even more recently [14].

On the basis of these considerations, and using M-mode echocardiography, we set out to verify, in a small but select group of hypertensives, the effects on the dimensions and functions of the left ventricle brought about by the acute and chronic administration of an anti-hypertensive drug, Labetalol, which - according to pharmacological and clinical research - has a simultaneous alpha- and beta-blocking action.

Patients and method

The 15 patients studied were affected by uncomplicated essential hypertension classifiable (according to the WHO stages) as mild-to-moderate, aged between 40 and 65 years (average age 53 years). These 15 patients were selected on the basis of the exclusion of hypertensives with ischaemic heart disease, signs of cardiac insufficiency and in any case a cardiothoracic ratio of 50%. Many hypertensives were excluded from the trial because the echocardiographic examination was not considered technically optimal. Others, who had been accepted, were later deleted from the group owing to discontinuation of the drug. BP levels were measured with a sphygmomanometer and auscultation, after at least 5 minutes in the supine and 3 minutes in the upright position. Before accepting patients for the trial, a minimum of 3 BP readings taken on 3 nonconsecutive days was considered indispensable. All patients had been taken off treatment with any other anti-hypertensive drug at least 4 weeks before the commencement of the trial.

Labetalol was administered at an initial dose of 300 mg/day and increased gradually until the desired clinical result was obtained. The efficacious dose was 300-900 mg/day, (mean dose 500 mg/day). The clinical study was complemented with routine laboratory examinations, ECG and chest X-ray before and after the treatment period.

The ultrasound examination of the left ventricle, including a reference ECG and a carotidogram, was made before treatment, after 20 days of drug administration, and at the end of 2 months.

In a second phase of the trial, 8 of the patients were put onto Propranolol, instead of Labetalol, at sufficient doses to produce the same therapeutic effect. The efficacious dose of Propranolol varied between 80 and 240 mg. An echocardiographic examination of these patients was carried out 20 days and 2 months after commencement of the tratment.

Finally, 10 hypertensives not included in the study group were subjected to a clinical and echocardiographic assessment of the effect of an acute intravenous administation (fast bolus) of 50 mg of Labetalol. According to the same selection criterion with regard to the technical result of the echocardiogram, all other anti-hypertensive drugs were withdrawn from these patients at least 4 weeks before the trial began. The BP reading in the supine position was taken as the basal value, when stable for at least 20 min. BP, HR and echocardiograms were recorded before administration of the drug and 10, 20, and 30 minutes afterwards.

The echocardiogram was done with an Ekoline-20 (Smith-Kline) echocardiograph with an optical-fibre paper recorder and a paper speed of 100 mm/sec. A non-focused 2.25 MHz probe was used. The one-dimensional examination was done by laying the patient in a supine position, or in the left lateral decubital position with his trunk at a 30-45° angle to the horizontal plane and with a transducer placed in the 3rd-4th intercostal space on the left parasternum.

The measurements were taken after a point-base scan according to Feigenbaum. The measurements of the left ventricle were read at the level of the fragmentary echoes of the mitral valve. From the recordings obtained, the following parameters were studied:
- diastolic diameter (DSD) and systolic diameter (SSD) of the left ventricle;
- thickness of the interventricular septum and its excursion range;
- thickness, excursion range and maximum velocity of the posterior wall (Vmax);
- ejection time of the left ventricle.

These direct measurements provided the following quantitative data: percentage difference of systolic contraction (S%), mean velocity of circumference contraction (Vcf), ejection fraction (EF), and ventricular mass (VM).

Results

Acute administration: 50 mg by fast bolus i.v.

In the 10 patients studied, basal BP values were $196 \pm 24/114 \pm 14$. A reduction in systolic and diastolic BP was observed in all patients; the maximum decrease occurred within 10 min.; after 30 min. BP values were $164 \pm 29/103 \pm 18$ (with a reduction in comparison to basal values of $32 \pm 18/11 \pm 10$; $P < 0.01$). There was a very slight HR reduction (basal values 69.2 ± 14) reaching a maximum after 30 min. (- 3.7 n.s.).

DSD (basal values 5 ± 0.63) and SSD (basal values 3.2 ± 0.6) remained more or less unaltered (variations of 2%). Minimal changes were observed for Vcf (1.23 ± 0.4), Vmax of the posterior wall (4.46 ± 0.7) and S% (35 ± 3.5).

Chronic administration of Labetalol

The 15 patients who completed the trial had pre-treatment BP values of $172.6 \pm 10/110 \pm 8$. All registered a reduction in systolic and diastolic BP values (on the 20th day: $-15 \pm 17/14 \pm 8$, $P < 0.01$; after 2 months: $-19 \pm 15/18 \pm 12$, $P < 0.01$) so that the values observed after 60 days were $153.6 \pm 15/92.8 \pm 8$.

HR (pre-treatment values: 75 ± 13) was reduced after 20 days to 115 ± 8 (P 0.01); later, after 60 days, a slight but non-significant increase was detected, in comparison to the previous reading, but the values remained significantly lower than the basal ones (-8.3 ± -0.9; $P < 0.01$).

DSD (4.77 ± 0.41) and SSD (3.26 ± 0.56) remained virtually unchanged. Vcf reductions from 1.18 before treatment to 1.11 after 20 days (-6%) and to 1.03 after 60 days (-12,7%) were not significant.

The Vmax of the posterior wall (4.42 ± 0.78) remained practically unaltered and $\Delta S\%$ (33.2 ± 6.8) was reduced after 2 months by 0.9 (n.s.). Left ventricular mass (176 ± 31 gr), septum thickness (1.14 ± 0.12) and posterior wall thickness, the excursion range of the septum and of the posterior wall (0.95 ± 0.10) proved unchanged in comparison to the basal values (Fig. 1).

Comparative results of chronic administration of Propranolol-Labetalol

In the 8 patients treated first with Labetalol and then with Propranolol, basal mean BP values were $174 \pm 15/109 \pm 8$. A comparable therapeutic effect was achieved with average daily doses of 471 mg of Labetalol and 137 mg of Propranolol (BP after Labetalol: $147 \pm 13/88.5 \pm 9$; after Propranolol: $152 \pm 12/89 \pm 8$).

HR (basal values: 76.5) after Labetalol fell

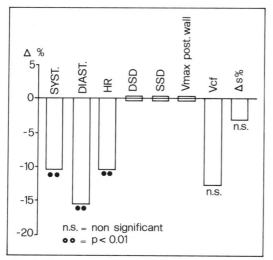

Fig. 1. Percentage variations (Δ%) in BP, HR and the echocardiographic parameters after 60 days' oral administration of a therapeutically efficacious dose of Labetalol.

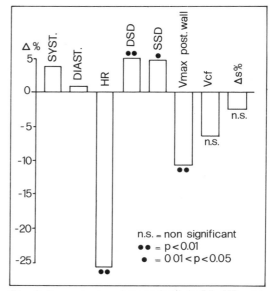

Fig. 2. Percentage variations (Δ%) in BP, HR and the echocardiographic parameters after 60 days' oral treatment with an equivalent dose of propranolol.

to 70.7 and after Propranolol to 52 (the decrease in HR as between the first and second drug was 18.5 ± 6.7; $P < 0.01$).

The basal mean DSD value was 4.85 ± 0.35; after treatment with Labetalol it was 4.90 ± 0.47 and 5.15 ± 0.38 after Propranolol (the DSD increase between the two drugs was checked in all patients: mean values 0.25 ± 0.16; P 0.01). Mean pre-treatment SSD was 3.22 ± 0.63; 3.30 ± 0.60 after Labetalol and 3.45 ± 0.50 after Propranolol (the increase between the two drugs occurred in 7 of the 8 patients: mean value 0.15 ± 0.13; P 0.05, 0.01). Pre-treatment Vcf was 1.21 ± 0.13; after Labetalol 1.08 ± 0.18; after Propranolol 1.01 ± 0.15 (the decrease between the two drugs was 0.07 n.s.).

The mean pre-treatment value of ΔS% (33.4 ± 6) remained more or less unchanged after Labetalol (-0.9) - a totally insignificant variation. Vmax of the posterior wall (mean pre-treatment values: 4.4 ± 0.8) dropped to 4.3 ± 1 after Labetalol and to 3.8 ± 0.9 after Propranolol (the decrease between the first and second drug was 0.47 ± 0.46; $P < 0.05$) (Fig. 2).

Remarks

This study examined the effects brought about on left ventricle size and function (by means of M-mode echocardiography) by the acute and chronic administration of a therapeutically efficacious dose of Labetalol. The 10 patients given 50 mg i. v. (fast bolus) of Labetalol, along with the decrease in supine BP, showed a considerable stability in HR and a possibility of overlap, in relation to basal values, of the internal dimensions of the left ventricle (DSD, SSD) and of the functional parameters (Vcf; S%; Vmax of the posterior wall). The anti-hypertensive action achieved by acute administration may be ascribed to the alpha-blocking component since by this route there is no beta component. The echocardiographic examination of the left ventricle does not reveal the modifications normally recorded after the administration of vasodilatory drugs (increase in HR; decrease in the internal dimensions of the left ventricle; increase in Vcf values, S%, Vmax of the posterior wall).

It seems therefore reasonable to suppose that the anti-hypertensive alpha component is opposed in its potential hyperkinetic effects on the heart by the beta-blocking component. The chronic oral administration of Labetalol in a group of patients with uncomplicated hypertension brought about a modest but significant decrease in HR after 2 months' treatment. The internal dimensions of the left ventricle (DSD, SSD) and the functional indices (Vcf, S%, Vmax of the posterior wall) proved to be substantially unaltered after administration of the drug (the reduction in Vcf was not statistically significant). In our chosen group of hypertensives, Labetalol did not therefore alter left ventricular function and dimensions, according to the echocardiographic study.

The thickness of the septum and the posterior wall and ventricular mass remained unchanged. However, in this regard, it is worth clarifiyng that the parameters concerned were already within the normal ranges in their basal conditions (only the thickness of the septum touched maximum normal levels) and in any case could undergo variations only after long periods of anti-hypertensive treament. It is not possible to add, on the basis of the echocardiagraphic criterion alone, a qualitative opinion on the subject of the finer mechanism of the drug action in its two parts to the quantitative opinion concerning the non-modification of left ventricular size or function after the administration of Labetalol. The attempt to draw any conclusions from the comparison of the clinical-echocardiographic results of Labetalol and Propranolol appears more difficult. In the 8 patients treated for the first 2 months with Labetalol and then with Propranolol, an overlapping therapeutic response was obtained for both supine and upright BP.

In comparison with Labetalol, Propranolol determines a highly significant decrease in HR, and the internal dimensions of the left ventricle, especially the telediastolic diameter, are increased. Vcf decreases very moderately; Vmax of the posterior wall decreases significantly but remains within normal limits. Whilst a different action on inotropism cannot be excluded, the overall critical examination of the results lends greater plausibility to the hypothesis that the most important quantitative modifications brought about by Propranolol may be attributed to the more consistent decrease in HR. The percentage of systolic contraction of the ventricular diameter (S%) appears substantially unchanged after Propranolol, suggesting that the increase in diastolic dimensions may be due to the slowing of HR while the reduction in Vcf (even if insignificant) may be due to the increase in ejection time.

On the other hand, this hypothesis is confirmed by recent literary data on the chronic use of Propranolol in subjects with normal LV function and dimensions [21, 22].

The (M-mode) echocardiographic method seems to be a sensitive and reproducible way of studying the effect of drugs on LV dimensions and functions. Even more useful in the assessment of acute administrations and individual doses of drugs, it has been directed largely towards the study of the systolic phase but, more recently, it has also produced encouraging results in the analysis of the diastolic phase [23].

Besides the optimal technical level of the recordings, the reliability of the method should lie in the use only of linear measurements revealed by the echocardiogram of the left ventricle. The internal telediastolic and telesystolic dimensions; the thickness, range and rate of excursion of the septum and of the posterior wall; the rate of circumference contraction (Vcf) and the systolic contraction of the internal diameter (S%); these are the parameters which are best suited to verifying the variations brought about by the drugs in ventricular performance and dimensions in subjects with symmetrical contraction of the walls.

Furthermore, in those patients with local contraction abnormalities, the echocardiographic method — which is not accurate for determining overall performance — may nevertheless be useful for evaluating the variations in local motility due to drugs.

References

1. Feigenbaum H.: *Echocardiography*, pp. 297-340, Philadelphia, Lea Febiger. 1976.
2. Popp R.L., Harrison D.C.: Ultrasonic cardiac echo-

graphy for determining stroke volume and valvular regurgitation. *Circulation*, 41, 493, 1970.

3. Pombo J. F., Troy B. L., Russel R.O. Jr.: Left ventricular volumes and ejection fraction by echocardiography. *Circulation*, 43, 480, 1971.

4. Fortuin N. J. , Hood W. P., Sherman M. E., et al.: Determination of left ventricular volumes by ultrasound. *Circulation*, 44, 575, 1971.

5. Troy B. L., Pombo J., Rackley C. E.: Measurement of left ventricular wall thickness and mass by echocardiography. *Circulation*, 45, 602, 1972.

6. Teichlolz L. E., Kreulen T., Herman M. V., et al.: Problems in echocardiographic volume determinations: Echocardiographic correlations in the presence or absence of asynergy. *Amer. J. Cardiol.*, 37, 7, 1976.

7. Mason S. J., Fortuin N. J.: L'uso dell'ecocardiografia per la valutazione quantitativa della funzione ventricolare sinistra. *Progr. in Patol. Cardiovasc.*, 3, 308, 1980.

8. Burgraaf G. W., Parker J. O.: Left ventricular volume changes after amyl nitrite and nitroglycerine in man as measured by ultrasound. *Circulation*, 49, 136, 1974.

9. Redwood D. R., Henry W. L., Epstein S. E.: Evaluation of the ability of echocardiography to measure alterations in left ventricular volume. *Circulation*, 50, 901, 1974.

10. De la Calzada C. S., Ziady G. M., Hardarson T., et al.: Effect of acute administration of propranolol on ventricular function in hypertrophic obstructive cardiomyopathy measured by non-invasive techniques. *Br. Heart. J.*, 38: 798, 1976.

11. Winkle R. A., Goodman D. J., Popp R. L.: Echocardiographic evaluation of propranolol therapy for mitral valve prolapse. *Br. Heart. J.*, 38, 126, 1976.

12. Hirshleifer J., Crawford M., O'Rourke R. A., et al.: Influence of acute alterations in heart rate and systemic arterial pressure on echocardiographic measures of left ventricular performance in normal human subjects. *Circulation*, 52, 835, 1975.

13. Cherchi A., Fonzo R., Lai C., Mercurio G., Bina P., Cioglia G.: Effetto della nifedipina sulle dimensioni ecocardiografiche del ventricolo sinistro nella cardiopatia ischemica: confronto con placebo, propranololo e trinitroglicerina. Atti del Simposio Internazionale su: *Esperienze cliniche con nifedipina.* Rome, Cepi, 1979.

14. Savage D. D., Drayer J. I. M., Henry W. L., Mathews E. C., Ware J. H., Gardin J. M., Coher E. R., Epstein S. E., Laragh J. H.: Echocardiographic assessment of cardiac anatomy and function in hypertensive subjects. *Circulation*, 59, 623, 1979.

15. Brittain R. T., Levy G. P.: A Review of the animal pharmacology of labetalol, a combined α- and β-adrenoceptor blocking drug. *Br. J. Clin. Pharmacol.*, 3, 681, 1976.

16. Richards D. A.: Effetto del blocco combinato sui recettori alfa e beta adrenergici del labetalolo nell'uomo. pp. 20-28. In: *Atti Conv. Int. Ipertensione: Nuove prospettive terapeutiche.* Venezia, 18-20 Maggio 1978. Glaxo Italia 1978, 269.

17. Koch G.: Effetti emodinamici del blocco alfa e beta-recettoriale acuto con somministrazione di labetalolo e.v. e variazioni in corso di trattamento orale protratto in pazienti affetti da ipertensione essenziale. pp. 65-70. In: *Atti Conv. Int. Ipertensione: Nuove prospettive terapeutiche.* Venezia, 18-20 maggio 1978. Glaxo Italia 1978, 269.

18. Alicandri C. L., Agabiti-Rosei E., Fariello R., Corea L., Muiesan G.: Effetti emodinamici della somministrazione acuta e cronica di labetalolo nell'ipertensione arteriosa. pp. 31-39. In: *Atti Conv. Int. Ipertensione. Nuove prospettive terapeutiche.* Venezia, 18-20 maggio 1978. Glaxo Italia 1978, 269.

19. Condorelli M., Brevetti G., Chiariello M., De Caprio L., Lavecchia G., Paudice G., Rengo F.: Diagnostica incruenta nella valutazione clinica di un nuovo farmaco antiipertensivo. pp. 55-64. In: *Atti Conv. Int. Ipertensione: Nuove prospettive terapeutiche.* Venezia, 18-20 maggio 1978. Glaxo Italia 1978, 269.

20. Fagard R., Amery A., Reybrouk T., Lijnen P., Billiet L.: Response of the systemic and pulmonary circulation to alpha- and beta-receptor blockade (labetalol) at rest and during exercise in hypertensive patients. *Circulation*, 6, 1214, 1979.

21. Port. S., Cobb F. R., Jones R. H.: The effect of propranolol on left ventricular function in normal man. *Circulation*, 61, 358, 1980.

22. Crawford M. H., LIndenfeld J. A., O'Rourke R. A.: Effects of oral propranolol on left ventricular size and performance during exercise and acute pressure loading. *Circulation* 61, 549, 1980.

23. Zardini P. Gastaldi L., Cottino A. M., Forni B., Morello M., Uslenghi E.: L'ecocardiografia nella valutazione degli effetti farmaco-terapeutici. Atti del XIII Corso Cardiologico, Centro De Gasperi; Rome, Pozzi, 1980.

Hypertension, recent advances and research
edited by M. Condorelli, A. Zanchetti
Cortina International, Verona 1982

Vasodilatory drugs in the treatment of essential hypertension

P.F. ANGELINO, G.C. LAVEZZARO, M. BURAGLIO

Department of Cardiology, St. John the Baptist's Hospital, Turin (Italy)

Key words. Essential Hypertension; Vasodilator Drugs; Chronic Treatment; Hydralazine; Propyldazine; Cadralazine; Minoxidil; Prazosin; Labetalol; Calcium Antagonists; Verapamil; Nifedipine; Captopril, Indapamide; Guancydine; Bupicomide; Trimazosin; Prizidilol.

Summary. The paper presents a description of the therapeutic properties of the vasodilators used in the chronic treatment of arterial hypertension.
The following are described with reference to each drug: the action mechanism, the dosage, indications, contraindications (if any), and side effects.
The first drug described is Hydralazine, followed by some drugs still in the experimental stage (Propyldazine and Cadralazine).
The study proceeds with a description of the potent Minoxidil, and then Prazosin.
The paper also covers Labetalol, the calcium antagonists and Captopril, which have an anti-hypertensive effect also through vasodilation although they are not pure vasodilators.
Lastly, some drugs only recently discovered and used are described: Indapamide, Guancydine, Trimazosin and Prizidilol.
We report on our own clinical and experimental experience with many of the drugs.

Introduction

For the treatment of primary hypertension, a disease with a multi-factorial pathogenesis, the drugs available have a variety of action mechanisms. Their association leads to better therapeutic results, with fewer side effects.

Whatever the factors bringing about arterial hypertension, the final pathogenetic moment always consists in an increase in the peripheral resistances. Drugs which reduce these peripheral resistances should constitute the ideal remedy in the treatment of hypertension.

But the isolated and long-term use of such drugs is limited by at least 3 factors:
1) reflex stimulation of sympathetic activity through secondary action on the baroreceptors on reduction of blood pressure, and through direct action on the central nervous system brought about by the high angiotensin levels;
2) increased PRA (plasma renin activity);
3) sodium and water retention which, combined with increased sympathetic activity, leads to an increased stroke volume which limits its hypotensive effect.

The drugs best associated with the vasodilators are those beta-blockers which oppose sympathetic stimulation and increased PRA, and diuretics which counteract sodium and water retention.

Leaving aside the parenteral use of potent vasodilators, which are used successfully in hypertensive emergencies (sodium nitroprusside, diazoxide, phentolamine, trimethaphan camphorsulfonate), let us concentrate on the oral vasodilators which are suitable for long-term administration.

According to the numerous haemodynamic studies, the vasodilators can be divided into two groups on the basis of the simultaneous presence or otherwise of dilation of the capacitance vessels, i.e. of the venular system. This is of special clinical importance in that the vasodilators which do not cause the dilation of the venous bed bring about an increase in stroke volume which operates against the reduction in blood pressure and may provoke angina and sometimes even cardiac decompensation.

The vasodilatory drugs which act on both the veins and arteries are devoid of such unpleasant side effects.

We shall now consider the different vasodilators, describing their main characteristics, any contraindications and the advantages to be obtained from each drug.

Hydralazine

The fundamental action mechanism of this drug in bringing about a decrease in blood pressure lies in a myorelaxing action aimed at the peripheral arterioles [1, 2, 3].

The dilatory action is much greater on the resistance vessels than the capacitance vessels [1, 2, 3, 4].

The isolated use of hydralazine leads to a hyperdynamic stimulation which may destroy instable cardiovascular equilibriums.

The vasodilatory action varies, and it increases plasma flow in the kidney, brain, spleen and around the heart, whilst plasma flow at muscle-skin vessel level is not significantly changed, indeed it is often reduced [1, 2, 4].

This drug must be used with caution in patients suffering from coronary diseases and in carriers of severe mitral stenosis. It has certain side effects, some of which appear at the beginning of treatment and others later on. Among the early side effects we draw attention to: headache, nausea, vomiting, tachycardia, dizziness, muscular weariness, sleepiness, diarrhea or constipation, paresthesia and angina. We also point out that these effects may be transitory [5, 6, 7, 8, 9] and in any case may be eliminated or at least minimized by the simultaneous use of diuretics, beta-blockers, or inhibitors of the sympathetic nervous system with a central action.

Side effects appearing later include: the lupus-like syndrome [10], arthralgia [11], fever.

Drugs of this category are mainly indicated for use in hypertensives with reduced renal function; in fact, it has been observed that the reduction in blood pressure in such patients is accompanied by improved renal function [12].

Propyldazine

Among the derivatives of hydralazine we recall propyldazine, a 3-hydrazino-pyridazine derivative, which, in studies carried out in both animals and man, has proved to possess a hypotensive action 5-13 times greater than hydralazine and a level of acute and chronic toxicity several times lower [13, 14, 15, 16].

The results we obtained with 20 serious hypertensives showed that propyldazine at the dose of 6 mg/day brought about a marked reduction in both systolic and diastolic blood pressure.

The mean blood pressure reduction obtained by adding propyldazine to beta-blockers and diuretics was 32 mmHg for systolic BP and 22 mmHg for diastolic BP [17]. The drug was well tolerated and, in particular, our patients did not experience tachycardia or sodium and water retention — probably because of the simultaneous administration of beta-blockers and diuretics.

Some patients complained of headache, at times severe, at the beginning of treatment with propyldazine, but this effect was always of brief duration, disappearing within a few days.

Creatinine clearance at the end of treatment showed a mean increase of 6 ml/min. and this increase was most significant in those patients with changes in the indices of renal function [17].

Cadralazine

Cadralazine is another derivative of hydralazine with a peripheral vasodilatory effect.

It begins to act gradually, not abruptly. Clinical research carried out in Switzerland and in our department has shown that the drug used at daily doses of 7.5-20 mg, together with beta-blockers and diuretics, is efficacious and well tolerated even with long-term administration [18, 19, 20].

According to our data, cadralazine administered alone at the dose of 10-20 mg/day possesses a considerable anti-hypertensive action and, furthermore, our study proved that, unlike the other drugs of this group, cadralazine does not cause sodium and water retention [20].

Minoxidil

Minoxidil is the most potent orally active vasodilator; it acts directly on arteriolar wall smooth muscle; it has no central action and no effect on the adrenergic nervous system.

Its action is rapid and long-lasting. It does not cause orthostatic hypotension but does lead to a marked retention of water and sodium.

This is in fact its most unpleasant drawback and the most difficult to counter, as it requires the simultaneous administration of high doses of diuretics which are often poorly tolerated by the patient.

Minoxidil was used in 14 patients with serious arterial hypertension who were particularly resistant to conventional anti-hypertensive drugs.

Blood pressure (pre-treatment values 249-149) fell to 141/88 after treatment with minoxidil.

Besides water retention, we also noted the appearance of hypertrichosis, in any case already described in other studies [21, 22, 23].

Throughout the trial period, which lasted an average of 6 months, blood pressure was kept within the normal range and there was no evidence of electrolytic changes, serum glucose increases, impaired liver function, increases in enzymes such as the transaminases, nor any coagulation defects. Nor was there a positive reaction to Coombs' test or the appearance of ANA.

An interesting finding concerns the behaviour of the renal clearances. In all cases in which these were reduced there was an improvement, and this improvement was especially marked in those patients whose renal filtrate was considerably reduced [21].

We have no experience of the treatment of anginous hypertensives with this drug, but recent publications show that, when associated with beta-blockers and diuretics, it may be used in such patients without risk [24].

It is our opinion that such drugs are best employed in the treatment of hypertensives who have not responded satisfactorily to previous treatment with beta-blockers and diuretics, or who reveal impaired renal clearances.

Prazosin

Prazosin, a quinoline derivative, is a new, orally active, anti-hypertensive drug.

Its precise action mechanism is unknown and the subject of much controversy.

It has a relaxing action on the smooth muscle of animals but in man it has, above all, a post-synaptic alpha-blocking action [25].

Unlike the other vasodilatory drugs, prazosin does not cause reflex tachycardia and does not increase PRA [26].

Like all alpha-blockers, it may cause orthostatic hypotension; the fall in blood pressure which accompanies the reduction in the peripheral resistances is not followed by a significant change in cardiac output, heart rate, renal plasma flow, and glomerular filtration rate [27].

In a study made by Pitts, prazosin alone was seen to reduce supine BP by 14/10 and upright BP by 18/14 [28].

Its efficacy is increased if used in association with beta-blockers and diuretics.

The initial dose may provoke syncope which occurs 30-60 minutes after the first administration [29]. It is therefore advisable that treatment should begin with a dose of 0.5 mg/day and that the patient be kept in a supine position.

Once the danger of syncope following the first administration has passed, treatment may be continued with doses of 1 mg three times a day, later increasing to up to 20 mg/day and more.

The side effects of the drug include postural dizziness, headache, fatigue, asthenia, nausea, vomiting, diarrhea. These side effects overlap with those induced by alpha-methyl-dopa.

Postural dizziness is the commonest side effect and was found in 13.7% of the patients studied [28]. In most cases, this effect disappears within a few days, but at times it persists and the treatment has to be suspended. The laboratory analyses revealed no haematological, renal, liver or other impairments.

Considering its efficacy in reducing the after-load, without increasing the venous return flow or causing tachycardia, prazosin may be considered a highly suitable drug for the treatment of hypertension in patients tending to show cardiac insufficiency.

Labetalol

Labetalol differs from the other common drugs which block the adrenoceptors in that it blocks both the alpha- and beta-receptors [30].

The use of phentolamine, a pure alpha-blocker, was tested in the treatment of hypertension, but some effect is obtained only at high doses, with side effects so great as to make its chronic administration impossible [31].

Phentolamine was later used in association with a beta-blocker, to counteract the reflex effects, and good results were obtained, from the point of view of tolerance and in terms of the hypotensive response [32, 33, 34].

The use of the beta-blockers, whilst inducing a decrease in blood pressure, at least in the early treatment period causes an increase in the peripheral resistances; hence the importance of the association of beta-blocker and vasodilator (in this case an alpha-blocker) to obtain the combined pharmacological mechanism of the 2 drugs.

In the light of the above considerations, the interest aroused by a drug like Labetalol is obvious: it can develop both alpha-blocking - and therefore potentially vasodilatory - and beta-blocking activity in the same molecule.

A haemodynamic study after treatment for 4 weeks with fixed doses (800 mg) of Labetalol, revealed that cardiac output during rest was unchanged, whilst peripheral resistances during rest were reduced (-18%) [35].

A study of ours [36] shows that the reduction in both systolic and diastolic BP is maintained even under work load. The determination of the blood pressure values under work load controlled on the cycloergometer, confirming the reduction in the peripheral resistances, showed that the control of blood pressure values is particularly valid for diastolic BP. We believe that Labetalol represents a real advantage in the long-term treatment of arterial hypertension in that, thanks to its balanced effect on the alpha- and beta-receptors, it reduces the possible side effects arising from the blockade of the alpha- or beta-receptors alone, at the same time preserving the heart-protecting properties of the beta-blockers.

Owing to the simultaneous vasodilatory effect, Raynaud's phenomena are not observed.

With regard to hypertensives with concomitant pathologies, the drug is particularly suitable for subjects with peripheral vascular disease, or coronary heart diseases, and even in those who have already suffered vascular brain damage.

The decrease in blood pressure is accompanied by a reduction in neither the glomerular filtrate [37] nor the cerebral flow [38], and cardiac performance is improved [39].

It is shown that hypertensive drop-out is in direct proportion to the number of drugs which the patient must take daily, as well as to the side effects of the drugs. Therefore, the use of a single drug with alpha- and beta-blocking properties does not require combined treatment with a vasodilatory drug, thus reducing the number of drugs to be taken. Furthermore, a balanced action on the alpha- and beta-receptors is better tolerated by the patient.

Orthostatic hypotension is rare with Labetalol: other side effects of the drug may be gastro-intestinal symptoms, dyspnea, fatigue and dizziness [40]. These side effects are also defined as the "adaptation crisis" and are, moreover, of slight proportions and limited to the beginning of the treatment.

Calcium antagonists

Recently a new category has been added to the hypotensive-vasodilatory drugs: the calcium antagonists, which had already long been used in the treatment of angina and in cases of arrhythmia [41, 42].

The contraction of smooth muscle fibre is Ca-dependent and cannot be brought about on isolated smooth muscle fibre unless Ca ions are present in the solution [43, 44]. Ca ions are needed in the smooth muscle fibres together with Na ions for the electrogenesis of the action potentials, as carriers of depolarizing electric charges into the cell. Drugs which reduce the availability of Ca ions for the muscular contraction mechanism reduce the contraction and therefore, at the level of vascular wall smooth muscle, give rise to vasodilation [45].

The use of these drugs (Verapamil, Nifedipine) in the treatment of arterial hypertension significantly reduces systolic and diastolic blood pressure in both the supine and upright positions.

This decrease is not accompanied by increased heart rate, cardiac inotropism, or significant increases in PRA, factors which have already been shown to render eventually inefficacious the therapeutic results which may be obtained by the isolated use of a vasodilatory drug.

The use of these drugs does not provoke either headache or palpitations, and rarely flushing. Oedema may appear in the lower limbs due to the arteriolar vasodilatory effect which is not accompanied by an equivalent dilation of the venous bed. The action of Ca-antagonist drugs on the inotropic effect of the myocardium must also be considered. The ideal anti-hypertensive drug should be capable of reducing peripheral resistances without diminishing the strength of the myocardium, with the exception of cases of hyperkinetic hypertension where the decrease in the contractile force is beneficial.

The Ca ions are also necessary for the electromechanical coupling of the myocardiac fibre.

Fleckenstein's studies [46], however, have proved that the Ca-antagonist drugs have a greater affinity for the smooth muscle cells of the vessels than for those of the myocardium.

Furthermore, Grun et al. [45] noted that the Ca-antagonists have a vasodilatory effect on the arteries at lower dosages than that which blocks the effects of glucoside on the myocardium.

In other words, the ventricular myocardium treated with glucosides is somewhat insensitive to the negatively inotropic action of the Ca-antagonists at the dosage used in the anti-hypertensive treatment. The positively inotropic action of the glucosides is therefore preserved when Ca-antagonist drugs are used as anti-hypertensives.

In short, we consider the Ca-antagonist drugs an excellent remedy for arterial hypertension, especially when the hypertensive condition is accompanied by angina or arrhythmia.

In any case, we recommend that they be used with caution in the presence of latent or evident myocardiac insufficiency, which will always require combined therapy with cardiokinetic drugs.

Indapamide

Indapamide is a non-thiazide chlorosulfamide derivative with an indolic nucleus. It has recently been introduced on the market for the treatment of hypertension, on which it acts by reducing the peripheral vascular resistances [47]. Its action mechanism is based on the reduction in the contractility of the smooth muscle cells of the vascular wall, by normalizing the membrane ion exchanges and decreasing the response of noradrenalin and angiotensin to stimulation [48].

Our study was carried out on 20 male patients with moderate arterial hypertension.

Basal blood pressure was measured repeatedly in all patients and after 3-5 days they were subjected to the ergometric test. They were then administered 2.5 mg of indapamide versus placebo.

The hypotensive response of the systolic and diastolic blood pressure was evaluated after 30 days of treatment, both during rest and under work load; in the same way, heart rate values recorded in basal conditions were compared with those found during the ergometric test.

The results of this trial confirm the good therapeutic efficacy of indapamide in the treatment of moderate hypertension.

The decrease in systolic blood pressure, already significant in basal conditions, remains constant during physical esercise. But the more important results are those obtained for diastolic blood pressure during rest and effort.

Whereas the proportions of the decrease remain more or less constant at medium-low loads, it becomes more marked as the effort increases until almost normal values are reached (89 ± 5.68 mmHg at the 3rd phase; 92.5 ± 7.58 mmHg at the 4th phase) [49].

These results are in conformity with theoretical suppositions and previous studies in confirming that the anti-hypertensive action of indapamide is based above all on the reduction of the peripheral resistances. This action becomes even more significant during effort when the vasodilatory effect produced by muscular exercise is complemented by the pharmacological effect of indapamide which operates even in conditions of particular stress on the cariovascular apparatus.

To sum up, indapamide acts on systolic and, especially, diastolic blood pressure, both in the supine and upright positions, and does cause orthostatic hypotension. It is very well tolerated, does not modify blood pressure in normotensives, acts at a low dosage (2.5 mg/day) and requires only one daily administration. Furthermore, its therapeutic effect is of long duration, without needing to increase the dose.

Captopril

Captopril (SQ 14,225; D-3-mercapto-2-methyl-propanoyl-1-proline) is an anti-hypertensive compound taken orally which acts primarily as an inhibitor of the converting enzyme (Angiotensin-Converting Enzyme, ACE). Consequently, Captopril blocks the pressor effect of angiotensin I [50] but not that of angiotensin II [51]; moreover, since the converting enzyme may be identified as kininase II, an enzyme which hydrolyzes the bradykinin, the administration of Captopril also leads to an increase in plasma kinin levels [52, 53, 54].

The drug was first proposed for the treatment of hypertension accompanied by high plasma renin activity (PRA), i.e. where a hyperproduction of angiotensin II could be expected [55]. Recently it has been shown that it is also effective in patients with normal or low PRA. The action mechanisms of the drug cannot therefore be attributed solely to the suppression of angiotensin II [56, 57, 58, 59].

Our study [60] was carried out on 19 patients suffering from serious hypertension who had not responded adequately to conventional drugs, even at high dosages.

After a wash-out period of at least 15 days, these patients were given Captopril at dosages ranging from 100 to 400 mg/day. If blood pressure did not return to normal with 400 mg, Chlorthalidone or Furosemide at the dose of 50 mg/day was added.

Blood pressure was reduced in all patients with Captopril but values were not always normalized, until a diuretic was added. Mean blood pressure, initially 152 ± 16 mmHg supine and 146 ± 12 upright, was reduced with Captopril to 127 ± 15 and 124 ± 12 respectively, and further decreased, to 106 ± 10 and 101 ± 9, after the addition of the diuretic.

Captopril was therefore shown to be an anti-hypertensive drug capable of reducing systolic and diastolic blood pressure in both the supine and upright positions.

This finding is of particular importance given that the patients were serious hypertensives who had not responded satisfactorily even to high dosages of conventional anti-hypertensive drugs, dosages which in most cases could not be increased on account of intolerable side effects.

Blood pressure is reduced gradually and, as other authors have found, no relationship was observed between pre-treatment PRA levels and the hypotensive response [53, 54, 61]. The fact that low and normal PRA subjects, as well as high PRA patients, responded to Captopril proves that the mechanism through which the hypotensive effect operates cannot be attributed esclusively to the conversion of angiotensin I into angiotensin II [56, 57, 58, 59].

It would therefore seem possible to confirm the hypothesis already put forward by other authors that the inhibition of the converting enzyme brings about an increment in the kinin pool, which may thus have a direct vasodilatory effect at the level of the arterioles and the effect of stimulating the renal release of prostaglandins with a vasodilatory action [56, 62, 63, 64, 65, 66, 67].

Besides inhibiting the formation of angiotensin II, this drug also has a vasodilatory action. It has few or no side effects. We observed only one case of ageustia, and one case of skin rash which promptly receded when the Captopril dose was reduced. There were no significant changes in erythrosedimentation, hemochrome, azotemia, serum protein, liver enzymes, prothrombin time, bilirubinemia, vanylmandelic acid and urinary catecholamines, ANA, urine test results or proteinuria. Unlike other authors [68], we did not notice pernicious leukopenia.

Some patients complained of asthenia, but this is to be considered an effect of the decrease in blood pressure rather than a direct effect of the drug.

Guancydine

Guancydine is a new anti-hypertensive drug which blocks the vasopressor response of angiotensin and reduces that of noradrenalin [69].

Freis and Hammer [70, 71] hold that it has an action similar to hydrazine, i.e. that it acts directly on the muscle of the vascular walls [70, 72]. The sympathetic reflexes are not blocked and therefore this drug brings about tachycardia and increased cardiac output.

Guancydine differs from hydralazine in that it causes dilation of both the capacitance and resistance vessels. Clinical studies on man have shown that the drug, at a dose of 100 - 500 mg/day, has a hypotensive effect [70, 72, 73]. Diastolic blood pressure undergoes a greater reduction with Guancydine than with Hydralazine [71].

It causes a very pronounced fluid retention

[71, 73], but gives rise to headache less often than Hydralazine.

Other side effects are: postural dizziness, palpitations, epigastric pains, disorientation, hallucinations, vomiting, nausea, congestive cardiac insufficiency, paresthesia and depression [71, 74].

The clinical application of the drug is limited by water retention and tachycardia. These undesired effects can be overcome by the administration of diuretics and beta-blockers [71, 75].

The drug may be used instead of Hydralazine as the third drug for patients who have not responded satisfactorily to diuretics and adrenergic blockers.

Bupicomide

This is a new vasodilatory drug used in the treatment of mild hypertension.

Bupicomide, which inhibits dopamine beta-hydroxylase, lowers blood pressure by acting as a vasodilator, rather than by inhibiting the synthesis of noradrenalin [76].

Chrysant et al. [77], in a study of 10 male patients with mild-to-moderate hypertension, found that mean blood pressure was reduced from 165-100 to 159-95 mm/Hg.

This result was obtained with doses of between 125 and 625 mg every 8 hours. Blood pressure values are reduced by means of the reduction in peripheral vascular resistances through the dilation of the arterioles. The most marked side effects were headache and palpitations which were so intense that treatment had to be suspended. Other, lesser side effects were fatigue, sleepiness, confusion and flushing.

Trimazosin

Trimazosin is an oral hypotensive drug acting through peripheral vasodilation [78].

Vlachakis et al. administered doses of 300-500 mg for 14-16 weeks and obtained a significant reduction in systolic and diastolic BP values in both the supine and upright positions. Mean BP was reduced (upright) from 155/113 to 139/98 and (supine) by 23/14.

The drug is well tolerated and has few side

Table I.

Drug	Aterial res.	Venous cap.	Heart rate	H₂O Na Retention
Hydralazine	++	unchanged	++	+
Propyldazine	++	unchanged	+	+
Cadralazine	++	unchanged	+	/
Minoxidil	+++	unchanged	++	+++
Prazosin	+	unchanged	unchanged	/
Labetalol	++	unchanged	unchanged	/
Ca Antagonists	+	unchanged	—	unchanged
Indapamide	+	unchanged	unchanged	unchanged (—)
Captopril	+	unchanged	(+)	—
Guancydine	++	+	+	++
Bupicomide	+	unchanged	+	/
Trimazosin	+	/	/	/
Prizidilol	+	/	—	—+

effects: headache, sleepiness, restlessness, nausea, constipation, dizziness, reduced hearing, chest pain and abdominal pain [78, 79].

Prizidilol

Prizidilol is a new anti-hypertensive drug which has a pre-capillary vasodilatory action and a beta-blocking action.

The administration of this drug at the dose of 300-600 mg/day brings about a significant reduction in systolic and diastolic blood pressure in both the supine and upright positions. This reduction is not accompanied by any increase in heart rate, PRA or aldosterone.

It leads to moderate water retention and a modest increase in catecholamines [80].

References

1. Freis E.D., Rose J.C., Higgins T.F. et al.: The hemodynamic effects of hypotensive drugs in man. IV 1-hydrazinophthalazine. *Circulation*, 8, 199, 1953.
2. Ingenito A., Barrett, J., Procita L.: Centrally mediated peripheral hypotensive effects of reserpine and hydralazine when perfused through the isolated in situ cat brain. *J. Pharmacol. Exp. Ther.*, 170, 1969.
3. Craves B., Barrett H., Cameron H., Yonkman F.: The activities of 1-hydrazinophthalazine (Ba-5968), a hypotensive agent. *J. Amer. Pharmacol. Assoc. (Sci. Ed.)* 40, 1951.
4. Koch-Weser J.: Vasodilator drugs in the treatment of hypertension. *Arch. Intern. Med.* 133, 1974.
5. Moyer J. H.: Hydrallagin (Apresoline) hydrochloride,

pharmacological observation and clinical results in the therapy of hypertension. *Arch. Intern. Med.* 91, 1953.
6. Aenishanslin W., Pestalozzi-Kerpel J., Dubach U.C. et al.: Antihypertensive therapy with adrenergic beta-receptor blockers and vasodilators. *Eur. J. Clin. Pharmacol.* 4, 1972.
7. Schroeder H.A.: The effect of 1-hydrazinophthalazine in hypertension. *Circulation* 5, 1952.
8. Kellaway, G.S.M.: Adverse drug reactions during treatment of hypertension. Symposium on Hypertension. Drugs, 2 (Suppl. I) 91, 1976.
9. Hughes W. M., Dennis E., Moyer J. H.: Treatment of hypertension with oral reserpine alone and in combination with hydralazine or hexamethonium. *Am. J. Med. Sci.* 229, 1955.
10. Perry H.M. Jr., Schroeder, H.A., Conners P.: Abnormalities of circulating cells and proteins in hydralazine patients without toxic symptoms. *Am. J. Med. Sci.* 244, 1962.
11. Perry H.M. Jr., Schroeder H. A.: Syndrome-simulating collagen disease caused by hydralazine. *J.A.M.A.* 154, 1954.
12. Judson W. E., Hollander W., Wilkins R. W.: The effects of intravenous Apresoline (hydralazine) on cardiovascular and renal functions in patients with and without congestive heart failure. *Circulation* 31, 1956.
13. Carpi, C. et al.: *Toxicity and pharmacology studies on ISF 2123*, ISF Research Laboratories. Unpublished data.
14. Carpi, C., Dorigotti, L.: Antihypertensive activity of a new 3-hydrazinopyridazine derivative: ISF 2123. *Brit. J. Pharmacol.*, 52, 1974.
15. Dorigotti, L., Rolandi, R., Carpi, C.: A new antihypertensive compound: 3-hydrazino-6-(2-hydroxypropyl)-methylamino-pyridazine dihydrocloride (ISF 2123) *Pharm. Res. Com.* 8, 1976.
16. Garagnani, A., Faggioli, M., Lama, G.: Ricerche cliniche pilota sulla propildazina (ISF 2123) e sue asso-

ciazioni nell'ipertensione essenziale. *Arch. Med. Int.* 29, 1977.

17. Angelino, P.F., Lavezzaro, G., Carnovali, M.: Trattamento dell'ipertensione arteriosa grave con propildazina (ISF 2123) associata ad un diuretico e a un beta-bloccante. *Minerva Cardioangiol.* 27, 1979.

18. Van Brummelen, P., Buhler, F.R., Kiowski, W., Bolli, P., Bertel, O.: Antihypertensive efficacy of a new long-acting vasodilator ISF 2469, in combination with a beta-blocker and a diuretic. *Int. J. Clin. Pharmacol.* 17, 380, 1979.

19. Amann, F.W., Buhler, F.R.: Long-term antihypertensive therapy with a new vasodilator ISF 2469, in combination with a beta-blocker and a diuretic. *Clin. Europea* 6, 1028, 1979

20. Lavezzaro, G.C., Gastaldo, D., Noussan, P., Bensoni M., Parini, Angelino, P.F.: Effetti della Cadralazina (ISF 2469) sul bilancio idrosalino e sull'ipertensione essenziale. *Minerva Cardioangiol.* (in press).

21. Angelino P.F., Lavezzaro, G.C.: Trattamento dell'ipertensione arteriosa grave con un nuovo vasodilatatore periferico (Minoxidil) *Minerva Cardioangiol.* 27, 359, 1979.

22. Dormois, J., Young, J. L., Neiss, A.S.: Minoxidil in severe hypertension: value when conventional drugs have failed. *Am Heart. J.* 90, 3, 1975.

23. Mehta, P.K., Mamdani, B., Shansky, R.M., Mahurkar, S.D., Dunea G.: Severe hypertension treatment with Minoxidil. *J.A.M.A.* 233, 3, 1975.

24. Wilburn, R.L., Blaufis, A., Bennet, C.M.: Long-term treatment of severe hypertension with minoxidil, propranolol and furosemide. *Circulation*, 52, 706, 1975.

25. Pitkajarvi, T., Kyostula, S. et al.: Antihypertensive action of drug combination: Polythiazide, prazosin and tolamolol. *Curr. Therap. Res.*, 21, 751, 1976.

26. Kosman, M.E.: Evaluation of a new antihypertensive agent, prazosin hydrochloride (Minipress) *J.A.M.A.*, 238, 1977.

27. Koshy, M.C., Mullie, A. et al.: Physiologic evaluation of a new antihypertensive agent prazosin Hcl. *Circulation* 55, 1977.

28. Pitts, N.E.: The clinical evaluation of prazosin hydrochloride, a new antihypertensive agent. In: Cotton, D.W.K. (Ed.): *Prazosin — Evaluation of a new antihypertensive agent*, Proceedings of a Symposium held at the Interprofessional Centre, Genoa, 8 March 1974, Amsterdam Excepta Medica, 1974.

29. Stokes, G.S., Graham, R.M. et al.: Influence of dosage and dietary sodium on the first-dose effects of Prazosin *Br. Med. J.* 2, 1977.

30. Richards, D.A., Wooding, E.P. et al.: The effects of oral AH 5158, a combined alpha- and beta-adrenoceptor antagonist, in healthy volunteers. *Br. J. Clin. Pharmacol.* 1, 505, 1976.

31. Moyer, J.H., Caplovitz, C.: Clinical results of oral and parenteral administration of imidazoine hydrochloride (Regitine) in the treatment of hypertension and evaluation of the cerebral haemodynamic effects. *Am. Heart. J.*, 45, 602, 1953.

32. Beilin, L.J., Juel-Jensen, B.E.: Alpha- and beta-adre-

noceptor blockade in hypertension. *Lancet*, 1, 979, 1972.

33. Sannerstedt, R., Stenberg, J., Johnsson, G., Werko, L.: Haemodynamic interference of alprenolol with dihydralazine in normal and hypertensive man. *Am. J. Cardiol.* 28, 316, 1971.

34. Zacest, R., Gilmore, E., Koch-Weser J.: Treatment of essential hypertension with combined vasodilatation and beta-adrenoceptor blockade. *New Engl. J. Med.*, 268, 617. 1972.

35. Edwards R.C., Raftery, E.B.: Haemodynamic effects of long-term oral labetalol. *Brit. J. Clin. Pharmacol.*, Suppl. 3, 733, 1976.

36. Angelino, P.F., Marra, S.: Valutazione emodinamica del labetalolo mediante test da sforzo multistadio in pazienti con cardiopatia ischemica ipertensiva. *Nuove prospettive nella terapia dell'ipertensione*, Torino 17.4.1980

37. Maschio, G., E., Previato, G., Tessitore, N. Lupo, A., Loschiavo, C., Gammaro, L.: *Gli alfa e beta bloccanti nell'ipertensione*. Atti Convegno Taormina, 1979.

38. Martin, L.E., Hopkins, R., Bland, R, E.: Metabolism of labetalol by animals and man. *Brit. J. Pharmacol.*, Suppl. 3, 695, 1976.

39. Mancia, G., Zanchetti, A.: Studi effetti ipotensivi del Labetalol mediante registrazione continua pressione arteriosa. pp. 71-80. In: *Atti Conv. Int. Ipertensione: Nuove prospettive terapeutiche.* Venezia, 18-20 maggio 1978. Glaxo Italia 1978, 269.
International Congress on Hypertension, Venice, 1978.

40. Prichard, B.N., Richards, D.A. Proceedings of the second symposium on labetalol. *Br. J. Clin. Pharmac.*, 8, Suppl. 2, 85-244, 1979.

41. Phear, D.N.: Verapamil in angina: a double-blind trial. *Brit. Med. J.*, 2, 740, 1968.

42. Ekelund, L.G., Oro, L.: Anti-anginal efficiency of Adalat with and without a beta-blocker. A subacute study with exercise test. *III International "Adalat" Symposium* Amsterdam, Excerpta Medica, 218, 1974.

43. Fleckenstein, A.: Specific inhibitors and promoters of calcium action in the exercitation-contraction coupling of heart muscle and their role in the prevention of production of myocardial lesions. In: Harris P., Opie L. (Eds.) *Calcium and the heart.* London, Academic Press, 1970-1971.

44. Grun, G., Fleckenstein, A., Byon, K.Y.: Ca-antagonism, a new principle of vasodilatation *Proc. Internat. Physiol. Sci.* 9, 25, 221, 1971.

45. Grun, G. and Fleckenstein, A.: The electromechanical uncoupling of smooth vascular muscles as basic principle of coronary dilatation by nifedipine. *Arzneim-Forsch.*, 22, 334, 1972.

46. Fleckenstein, A., Grun, G., Byon, K.Y.: Gli effetti fondamentali calcio antagonisti del Verapamil sulle fibre miocardiche e sulle cellule muscolari lisce dei vasi. *Minerva Med*, 66, 1827, 1975.

47. Beregi, L.G.: Antihypertensive and saluretic properties of the indoline and iso-indoline series. *Current Med. Res. Opin.* 5, Suppl. 1, 1977.

48. Gargoul, Y.M., Mironneau, J.: Action de l'indapamide (1520 SE) sur la muscolature liss longitudinale de la

veine porte. *Current Med. Res. Opin.* 5, Suppl. 1, 1977.

49. Martiny, W., Ladetto, P.E., Lanzoni, M., De Berardinis, A., Riva, L., Angelino, P.F.: Valutazione con test ergometrico dell'efficacia terapeutica dell' indapamide. In press.

50. Ferguson, K.R., Brunner, H.R., Turini G.A. and Kinstru M.C.: A specific orally active inhibitoral angiotensin-converting enzyme in man. *Lancet*, 1, 775, 1977.

51. Murthy, V.S., Waldron, T.L., Goldberg, M.E. et al.: Inhibition of angiotensin-converting enzyme by SQ 14, 255 in conscious rabbits. *Eur. J. Pharmacol.* 46, 207, 1977.

52. William G.H., Hollenberg N.K.: Accentuated vascular and endocrine response to SQ 20, 881 in hypertension. *New Engl. J. Med.* 297, 184, 1977.

53. McCaa R.E., Hall J.E., McCaa C.S.: The effects of angiotensin-I-converting enzyme inhibitors on arterial blood pressure and urinary sodium excretion: rôle of the renal renin-angiotensin and kallikrein-kinin systems. *Cir. Res.* 43, 1-32, 1978.

54. Johnson A.R., Schulz W.W., Naguiera L.A., Erdos E.G.: Kinins and angiotensins. Angiotensin-I-converting enzyme (kininase II) in endothelial cells cultured from human pulmonary arteries and veins. *Clin. Exptl. Hypertension* 2, 659-674, 1980.

55. Case D.B., Wallace J.M., Keim H.J., Weber M.A., Sealey J.E., Laragh J.H.: Possible role of renin in hypertension as suggested by renin-sodium profiling and inhibition of converting enzyme. *New Engl. J. Med.* 296, 641, 1977.

56. Sullivan J.M., Ginsburg B.A., Ratts T.L., Johnson J.G., Barton B.R., Kraus D.H., McKinstry D.N., Muirhead E.E.: Hemodynamic and antihypertensive effects of Captopril, an orally active angiotensin-converting enzyme inhibitor. *Hypertension* 1, 4, 397, 1979.

57. Bravo E.L., Tarazi R.C.: Converting enzyme inhibition with an orally active compound in hypertensive man. *Hypertension* 1,1, 39, 1979.

58. Muirhead E.E., Prewitt R.L., Brooks B., Brasius W.L.: Antihypertensive action of the orally active converting enzyme inhibitor (SQ 14, 225) in spontaneously hypertensive rats. *Circ. Res.* 43 (Suppl. I), 1-53, 1978.

59. Mimran A., Targhetta R., Laroche B.: The antihypertensive effect of Captopril. Evidence for an influence of kinins. *Hypertension* 2,6, 732, 1980.

60. Lavezzano, G.C., Angelino, P.F., Gastaldo, D., Minelli, M., Paccotti, P., Angeli, A.: Trattamento dell'ipertensione arteriosa refrattaria con un farmaco inibitore dell'enzima convertente (Captopril). *Minerva Cardioangiol*, (in press).

61. Gavras, H. Brummer, H.R., Turini, G.A., Kezshaw, G.R. Tifft, C.P., Cattelod, D. Gavras, I., Unkovik R.A., McKinstug D.N.: Antihypertensive action of the oral angiotensin-converting enzyme inhibitor SQ 14, 225 in man. *New Engl. J. Med.* 298, 981, 1978.

62. McGill J.C., Hakovitz I.I.D., Lorragno A. et al.: Modulation and mediation of the action of the renal kallikrein-kinin system by prostaglandins. *Fed. Proc.* 35, 175, 1976.

63. McGill J.C., Nasilotti A.: Kinins, renal function and blood pressure regulation, *Fed. Proc.* 35, 172, 1976.

64. Damas J., Bourdon V.: Liberation d'acide arachidonique par la bradykinine. *Comptes Rendus*, 1445, 1974.

65. Murthy V.S., Waldron T.L., Coldberg M.E.: The mechanism of bradykinin potentiation after inhibition of angiotensin-converting enzyme by SQ 14, 255 in conscious rabbits. *Circ. Res.* (Suppl I): 1-40, 1978.

66. Bravo E.L., Tarazi R.C., Dustan H.P.: Multifactorial analysis of chronic hypertension induced by electrolyte-active steroids in trained, unanesthetized dogs. *Circ. Res.* 40 (Suppl. I): 1-40, 1977.

67. Cushman D.W., Cheung H.S.: Studies in vitro of angiotensin-converting enzyme of lung and other tissues. In: Genest J., Koiw E. (Eds.): *Hypertension*, Berlin, Springer-Verlag, 1972, p. 532.

68. Amann F.W., Buhler F.R., Conen D., Brunner F., Ritz R., Speck B.: Captopril-associated agranulocytosis. *Lancet*, 1, 150, 1980.

69. Cummings, J.R., Welter, A.M. et al.: Angiotensin-blocking actions of guancydine. *J. Pharmacol. Exp. Ther.* 170, 334, 1969.

70. Freis, E.D., Hammer J.: Guancydine, a new type of antihypertensive agent. *Med. Ann. D.C.* 38, 1969.

71. Hammer, J., Ulrych, M., et al.: Hemodynamic and therapeutic effects of guancydine in hypertension. *Clin. Pharmacol. Ther.* 12, 78, 1971.

72. Stembert, J., Sannerstedt, R. et al.: Hemodynamic studies on the antihypertensive effect of guancydine. *Europ. J. Clin. Pharmacol.* 3, 63, 1971.

73. Villareal, J., Arcila, H. et al.: Effects of guancydine on systemic and renal hemodynamics in arterial hypertension. *Clin Pharmacol. Ther.* 12, 838, 1971.

74. Clark D.W., Goldberg, L.I.: Guancydine; a new antihypertensive agent, used with quinethazone and guanethidine or propranolol. *Ann. Int. Med.* 76, 579, 1972.

75. Gilmore, E., Weil, J. et al.: Treatment of essential hypertension with a new vasodilator in combination with beta-adrenergic blockade. *New Engl. J. Med.* 282, 521, 1970.

76. Velasco, M., Gilbert, C.O. et al.: Comparative cardiovascular effects of hydralazine and a new antihypertensive agent, bupicomide (Abstract) *Circulation*, 50, 105, 1974.

77. Chrysant S.G., Adamopoulus P., et al.: Systemic and renal hemodynamic effects of bupicomide: a new vasodilator. *Am. Heart. J.* 93, 335, 1967.

78. Vlachakis N.D., Mendloroity, M. et al.: Treatment of essential hypertension with trimazosin, a new vasodilator agent. *Curr. Ther. Res.* 17, 564, 1975.

79. Unpublished data by McMahon F.G., Freis E.D. on file at Pfizer Central Research, Groton, Connecticut.

80. Fariello R., Alicandri C.L., Agabiti-Rosei E., Romanelli G., Castellano M., Beschi. M., Platto L., Leto S., Muiesan.: Effects of Prizidilol (SKF 92657) on blood pressure, haemodynamics, sympathetic nervous system activity and plasma volume in essential hypertension. Abstracts of: *Eighth Scientific Meeting of the International Society of Hypertension*, Milan, 1981.

Hypertension, recent advances and research
edited by M. Condorelli, A. Zanchetti
Cortina International, Verona 1982

Hypertension and coronary artery disease

E.A. SALCEDO

Cleveland Clinic Foundation, Cleveland, U.S.A.

Key words. Essential Hypertension; Coronary Artery Disease; Atherosclerosis.

Summary.   An analysis is made of the relationships between hypertension and coronary artery disease. Particular attention is devoted to the cause-and-effect relationship between systemic hypertension and the development of atherosclerosis especially with regard to the coronary arteries. Conversely, the authors also examine the inverse relationship, i.e. coronary artery disease as a possible cause of hypertension.

In considering the relationship between hypertension and coronary artery disease, two broad categorizations can be made. First, the impact of systolic and diastolic systemic hypertension on the development and progression of atherosclerosis in general and with regard to coronary artery disease in particular and second, coronary artery disease as a possible cause of hypertension.

The first consideration comes into focus with studies that are related to hypertension as a risk factor for coronary artery disease, and with the studies of the natural history of obstructive coronary artery disease where the most important factors in its progression can be evaluated.

When one considers the aspect of coronary artery disease as the cause of hypertension, the most important points to evaluate are the hypertensive response of the patients with coronary insufficiency, the hypertension seen in the early phases of myocardial infarction, and the possibile hypertensive responses in postcoronary bypass patients. A good understanding of these relations has practical repercussions that will help the clinician in dealing with patients with hypertension and coronary artery disease.

A. Hypertension as a risk factor for coronary artery disease

The importance of hypertension as a precursor of coronary artery disease events has been clarified with several prospective epidemiological and clinical reports. [1-9] The Framingham Study [5-9] is probably the best known of these reports and its scientific merit is well recognized. This has shown that without exception the risk of every major clinical manifestation of coronary artery disease is increased in hypertensives. This is true for any age and any sex. Blood pressure contributes to coronary disease incidence in proportion to the degree of hypertension, but the risk is at the same time greatly influenced by concomitant risk factors. Its contribution is, however, independent of all the other major risk factors. It also appears that hypertension is the most important identified contributor to coronary artery disease. The Framingham Study group has also asserted that both systolic and diastolic hypertension are of importance. Comparing subsequent cardiovascular disease in persons classified by their systolic versus diastolic pressure, there is nothing to suggest superiority of the diastolic pressure and that even isolated elevation of systolic pressure is important.

It is also relevant to consider the natural history of patients with known coronary artery disease and then to analyze the impact that hypertension has on their prognosis.

At the Cleveland Clinic, Dr. Proudfit [10] has followed for 10 years a large group of patients who had proven coronary artery disease by cardiac catheterization and who did not undergo revascularization surgery. In these patients, the most important prognostic factors in relation to survival were the number of arteries severely obstructed, significant involvement of the left ventricular function or ventricular aneurysm.

He also found that other prognostic influences at least partially independent of these factors were electrocardiographic evidence of left ventricular hypertrophy, diabetes and hypertension. In contrast to the Framingham Study, systolic hypertension seemed to have no significant effect on survivial but systolic and diastolic elevations had a definite adverse effect especially striking after 10 years' follow-up. On the other hand, Kramer et. al. [11] in studying patients by repeated catheterization, has found no significant influence of the usual risk factors, e.g. family history, cholesterol levels, diabetes, and hypertension in the progression of coronary artery disease.

B. Coronary artery disease as a cause of hypertension

Hypertensive responses are known to occur in the very early phase of acute myocardial infarction, with angina pectoris, and after certain forms of cardiac surgery such as coronary artery bypass grafting. These responses may all be related to a mass of neuroreceptor tissue lying just between the origin of the aorta and pulmonary artery and receiving blood supply from the proximal portion of the left coronary arteries. This has been proposed recently by James and collaborators [12].

The exact etiology of hypertension in the early phases of acute myocardial infarction is still speculative. It would be easy to attribute it to anxiety and stress with increased catechol release, but actually the type of hypertension often seen in these patients is frequently too severe to be readily attributable to emotions, diastolic levels sometimes being 160 mm. or more, and suggesting the presence of a special neuroreceptor within the heart itself.

A possibly related phenomenon may be the hypertension which is seen in patients after coronary artery bypass. At our institution Dr. Fouad has studied the hemodynamic and humoral characteristics of post-coronary-bypass hypertension in 85 patients demonstrating elevation of systemic vascular resistance and rapid heart rate without significant change in cardiac output [13]. There was an increase in systemic catecholamines suggesting a sympathetic overdrive. There was reduction in pressure with unilateral stellate block. These results suggest that post coronary bypass hypertension could be due to an afferent sympathetic reflux originating from the heart great vessels or coronary arteries.

References

1. Paul, O.: A survey of the epidemiology of hypertension: 1964-1974. *Mod. Concepts Cardiovasc. Dis.* 43, 99-102, 1974.
2. Kannel, W.B., Dawber T.R.: Hypertension as an ingredient of a cardiovascular risk profile. *Br. J. Hosp. Med.*, 508-524, 1974.
3. Sokolow, M., Perloff, D.: The prognosis of essential hypertension treated conservatively. *Circulation* 23, 697, 1961.
4. Lew, E.A.: Blood pressure and mortality: Life insurance experience, in: Stamler J., Stamler R., Pullman T.N.: *The Epidemiology of Hypertension.* New York, Grune & Stratton, 1967, p. 392.
5. Kannel, W.B., Gordon, T., Schwartz M.H.: Systolic vs. diastolic blood pressure and risk of coronary heart disease: The Framingham Study. *Am J. Cardiol.* 27, 335-346, 1971.
6. Kannel, W.B., Wolf, P.A., Verter, J., et. al.: Epidemiologic assessment of the role of blood pressure in stroke: The Framingham Study, *JAMA* 214, 301-310, 1970.
7. Kannel, W.B., W.P. Castelli, P.M. McNamara, et.al.: Role of blood pressure in the development of congestive heart failure: The Framingham Study. *New Engl. J. Med.* 287, 781-787, 1972.
8. Kannel, W.B., Shurtleff, D.: The natural history of arteriosclerosis obliterans. *Cardiovasc. Clin.* 3, 37-52, 1971.

9. Kannel, W.B., Dawber, T.R.: Hypertensive cardiovascular disease: The Framingham study, In G. Onesti, K.E. Kim, J.H. Moyer. *Hypertension: Mechanisms and Management*, New York, Grune & Stratton, 1973, pp. 93-110.

10. Proudfit, W.L., Bruschke, A.V., Sones, M.F.: Natural history of obstructive coronary artery disease: Ten-year study of 601 non-surgical cases. *Progress in Cardiovas. Disease* 21, 53-78, 1978.

11. Kramer, J.R., Matsuder, Y., Mulligan, J.C., Aranow, M., Proudfit, W.L.: "Progression of Coronary Atherosclerosis", *Circulation*, March 1981 (in press).

12. James, T.N., Hagerman, G.R., Orthaler, F.: Anatomic and physiologic considerations of a cardiogenic hypertensive chemoreflex. *Amer. J. Cardiol.* 44, 852, 1979.

13. Fouad, F.M., Estafanous, F.G., Bravo, E.L., Iyer, K.A., Maydak, J.H., Tarazi, R.C.: Possible role of cardiothoracic reflexes in postcoronary bypass hypertension. *Amer. J. Cardiol.* 44, 866, 1979.

Hypertension, recent advances and research
edited by M. Condorelli, A. Zanchetti
Cortina International, Verona 1982

Demonstration, by means of an acute haemodynamic study, of the beta-blocking effects of Labetalol in normotensive coronary heart disease patients

A. CHIDDO, D. MASTRANGELO, A. GAGLIONE, F. BOSCIA, D. QUAGLIARA, G. FRANCHINI, P. RIZZON

Department of Diseases of the Cardiovascular Apparatus, University of Bari

Key words. Labetalol i.v.; Haemodynamic Indices; Coronary Heart Disease; Left Ventricular Systolic Blood Pressure; Left Ventricular Telediastolic Blood Pressure; Aortic Diastolic Blood Pressure; Ejection Fraction; TSBP/TSV Ratio; Peripheral Alphalytic Action; Chronotropic Beta-blocking Action; Negative Inotropic Beta-blocking Action.

Summary.   The haemodynamic changes due to adrenergic blockade during Labetalol therapy (i.v.) were assessed in 15 normotensive coronary heart disease patients.
LVSBP, LVTDBP, AoDBP, E.F., the ratio TSBP/TSV, and other haemodynamic indices were evaluated.
We may therefore conclude that, in normontensive coronary heart disease patients, Labetalol exerts not only a peripheral alphalytic action but also an unquestionable chronotropic and negative inotropic beta-blocking action.

Labetalol is an anti-hypertensive drug with a special capacity for simultaneously blocking both alpha- and beta-adrenoreceptors. It is therefore in a position to bring about a substantial reduction in peripheral resistances without the occurrence of reflex effects such as tachycardia or orthostatic hypotension. Published studies on the subject underline essentially the importance of the alphalytic effect of the drug. These studies were conducted almost exclusively using non-invasive methods and, for obvious reasons, in hypertensive patients. The acute betalytic action of the drug, however, had not been demonstrated - at least, not in man - except indirectly using polygraphic or ergometric methods, which are unsuited to the purpose [1, 2]. On the other hand, an invasive study of 10 coronary heart disease patients (5 normotensive and 5 hypertensive), in whom left ventricular performance was assessed by means of the ejection fraction and the study of zonal kinetics, failed to reveal any negative inotropic effects produced by Labetalol [3].

The aim of this study was to assess the extent of the direct beta-blocking effect of the drug on the myocardium using systolic and diastolic indices of left ventricular performance considered as being relatively independent of peripheral haemodynamic alterations.

Patients and method

The present case study comprises a group of 15 patients, 14 male and 1 female, aged between 32 and 68 years (average age 49 years). All the patients were normotensive (aortic systolic BP 127 ± 18; aortic diastolic BP 74 ± 10) and had come in for observation with anginal disorders without any previous clinical history or ECG signs of infarction. For diagnostic purposes all the patients were subjected to right and left cardiac catheterization, left ventricular cinematography, aortography and selective coronarography.

Cardiac output was determined using the thermodilution method by means of a Swan-Ganz catheter introduced via a basilic vein. Complete right catheterization was performed by means of a Counrand catheter introduced via the same route. The left pressure readings were taken by means of the brachial insertion of a Millar Mikro-Tip catheter. The left ventricular cinematography (30° OAD projection) and the suprasigmoidal aortography (45° OAS projection) were effected using a monoplane angiograph with automatic injection of 45 cc. and 40 cc. respectively of iodate contrast (Urografin 75).

The following evaluations were made:
- heart rate (HR);
- left ventricular systolic blood pressure (LVSBP);
- left ventricular telediastolic blood pressure (LVTDBP);
- aortic diastolic blood pressure (AoDBP);
- dP/dT max.;
- Vmax (maximum theoretical fibre-shortening velocity at 0 load);
- left ventricular stress, obtained according to Mirsky's formula [4];
- left ventricular time, a time constant which characterizes the isometric relaxtion phase, as calculated according to Weiss's method [5].

The left ventricular telesystolic volume (TSV) and the left ventricular telediastolic volume (TDV) were calculated using Dodge's monoplane methods modified for 30° OAD projection. The ejection fraction (E.F.) was obtained by applying the following formula:

$$E.F. = \frac{TDV - TSV}{TDV} \%$$

As an index of ventricular performance in the diastolic phase, we also used the Kp or left ventricular chamber rigidity modulus [6] and the delta V/delta P ratio or overall compliance of the left ventricle. As regards the systolic phase, we calculated the instantaneous ratio between ventricular telesystolic blood pressure

and telesystolic volume (TSBP/TSV) [7], obtained, as in the case of the two previous indices, by synchronizing the left intraventricular pressure curve with the ventricular cinematography photograms. The TSBP/TSV ratio is independent of load conditions and gives a true picture of the inotropic modifications.

In addition, we assessed the effect of the drug on the peripheral arterial region and on the aorta by calculating the following indices:
- aortic time (AoT), a time constant which expresses the rate of the drop in AoDBP;
- the compliance of the arterial system (AoT/peripheral resistances);
- aortic impedance, obtained using MacDonald's angiographic method [8] according to the formula:

$$Z = \frac{c\,e}{\pi\,r^2}$$

(c = pulse wave velocity; $\pi\,r^2$ = area of aortic section; e = blood density).

The above-mentioned parameters were evaluated in basal conditions and 20 minutes after administration of a 3-minute intravenous injection of a 1 mg./Kg. dose of Labetalol. The examination was completed by selective coronarography performed via a retrograde brachial route according to the Sones technique.

Results and comment

The results of the study are given in Figs. 1, 2, 3, 4 and 5.

The non-increase in HR, in the presence of a reduction in peripheral resistances, LVSBP and AoDBP, is in itself evidence of a beta-blocking action of Labetalol sufficient to compensate for the secondary effects of the alpha-blockade. The increase in LVTDBP, albeit in the presence of a reduced parietal rigidity (reduced Kp and left ventricular time) and with virtually constant HR, may be ascribed to an increase in TDV and TSV. On the other hand, the increase in TSV and above all the clear-cut reduction in the TSBP/TSV ratio, an index which expresses the inotropic state regardless of peripheral modifications, would tend to indicate a reduction in inotropism as a

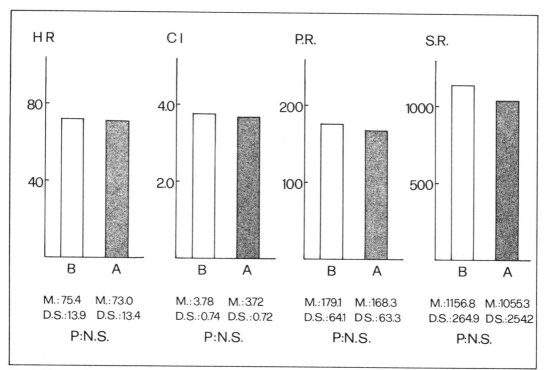

Fig. 1. Changes brought about by Labetalol in heart rate (HR), in cardiac index (CI), in pulmonary resistance (P.R.) and in systemic resistance (S.R.).

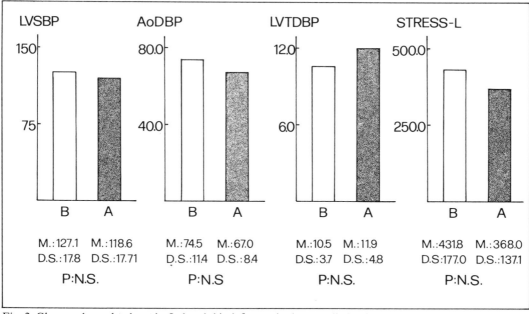

Fig. 2. Changes brought about by Labetalol in left ventricular systolic BP (LVSBP), in aortic diastolic blood pressure (AoDBP), in left ventricular telediastolic blood pressure (LVTDBP) and in left ventricular stress (Stress-L).

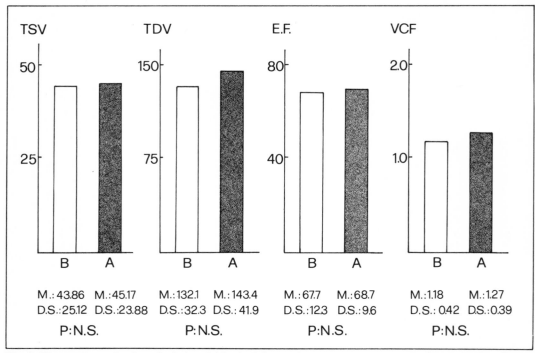

Fig. 3. Changes brought about by Labetalol in the left ventricular telesystolic volume (TSV), in the left ventricular telediastolic volume (TDV), in the ejection fraction (E.F.) and in the velocity of cardiac fibres (VCF).

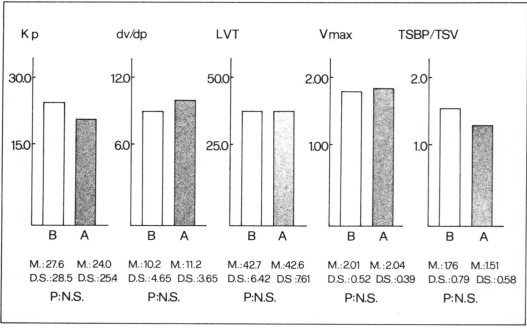

Fig. 4. Changes brought about by Labetalol in Kp, in the dV/dP ratio, in left ventricular time (LVT), in Vmax and in the TSBP/TSV ratio.

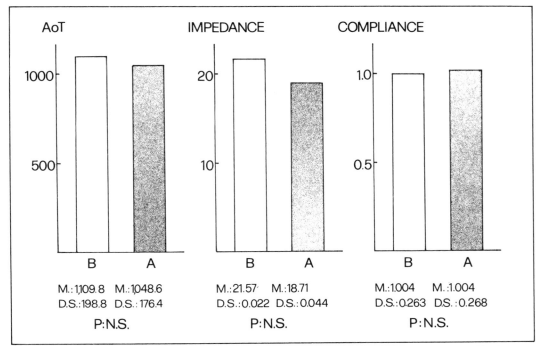

Fig. 5. Changes brought about by Labetalol in the aortic time (AoT), in the aortic impdance and in the compliance of the arterial sytem.

result of the beta-blockade. The Vmax, E.F. and VCF, contractility indices affected by afterload, show a tendency to increase, which, however, must be interpreted as a consequence of the reduction in peripheral resistances and not as an improvement in contractility.

We may therefore conclude that, in the normotensive coronary heart disease patient, Labetalol exerts not only a peripheral alphalytic action but also an unquestionable chronotropic and negative inotropic beta-blocking action.

References

1. Rossi, A., Ziacchi, V., Lomanto B.: Les intervalles de temps systoliques dans l'hypertension essentielle. *Arch. Mal. Coeur,* 72, 11, 1240-1246, 1976.
2. Cherchi, A., Fonzo, R., Lai, C., Mercurio, G.: Influenza del Labetalolo sul test di tolleranza allo sforzo in pazienti affetti da angina pectoris. pp. 40-54. In: *Atti Conv. Int. Ipertensione: Nuove prospettive terapeutiche.* Venezia, 18-20 maggio 1978. Glaxo Italia 1978, 269.
3. Trevi G.P., Benussi F., Dal Forno P., Franco G.F., Marini A., Sheiban I.: Modificazioni acute di parametri emodinamici e della cinetica zonale del ventricolo sinistro indotte dal Labetalolo in pazienti ipertesi anginosi. pp. 103-113. In: *Atti Conv. Int. Ipertensione: Nuove prospettive terapeutiche.* Venezia, 18-20 maggio 1978. Glaxo Italia 1978, 269.
4. Mirsky I.: Left ventricular stress in the intact human heart. *Biophys. J.* 9, 189, 1969.
5. Weiss J.L., Frederikson J.W., Weisfeldt M.L.: Haemodynamic determinants of the time course of fall in the left ventricular pressure. *J. Clin. Invest.* 58, 751, 1976.
6. Gaasch W.H., Levine H.J., Quinones M.A., Alexander J.K.: Left ventricular compliance: mechanisms and clinical implications. *Am. J. Cardiol.* 38, 645-653, 1976.
7. Suga H., Sagawa K.: Instantaneous pressure volume relationships and their ratio in the excised, supported canine left ventricle. *Circ. Res.* 35, 117-125, 1974.
8. MacDonald D.A.: *Blood flow in arteries.* London, Edward Arnold, 1974.

Hypertension, recent advances and research
edited by M. Condorelli, A. Zanchetti
Cortina International, Verona 1982

Chronic treatment of patients with essential hypertension and ischaemic heart disease with Labetalol: a clinical, ergometric and haemodynamic evaluation

A. STRANO, S. NOVO, L. SALERNO, G. LICATA, A. PINTO, G. DAVÌ, M. FAZIO

Institute of Clinical Medicine and Medical Therapy of University of Palermo
C.N.R.: Preventive Medicine Project - Hypertension Sub-project - University of Palermo
Institute of Medical Pathology "R", University of Palermo

Key words. Essential Hypertension; Ischaemic Heart Disease; Stable Angina Pectoris; Variant Angina Pectoris; Labetalol; Ergometer Test; Systemic Haemodynamics; Chest Pain Episodes; Nifedipine-Labetalol Association; Peripheral Haemodynamics; Rest Flow; Peak Flow; Systemic Vascular Resistances; Plasma Aldosterone; Plasma Renin Activity.

Summary The clinical, ergometric and haemodynamic effects of treatment with the alpha- and beta-adreno-receptor blocker Labetalol for 6 months were studied in 12 hypertensive patients with I.H.D., 6 males and 6 females, aged 40 to 70 years, with an average age of 54 ± 11.5 years.

Chronic treatment with Labetalol significantly reduced chest pain effort episodes and increased the angina threshold during the bicycle ergometer test in hypertensive patients with stable angina pectoris.

In two hypertensive patients with variant angina, a nifedipine-labetalol association (nifedipine 40 mg/die plus Labetalol 600 mg/die) noticeably improved spontaneous chest pain episodes.

Systemic systolic, diastolic and mean pressures were considerably reduced by Labetalol both at rest (supine and upright) and during exercise.

Systemic blood pressure was lowered by a reduction in systemic vascular resistances. In fact, heart rate was significantly reduced under all conditions (supine, upright and during exercise), but cardiac output was unchanged because of a rise in stroke volume which partially counterbalanced the reduction in pulse rate.

Rest flow and peak flow at the calf increased, and there was a parallel decrease in basal and minimal vascular resitances at the calf.

Postural hypotension was not observed after long-term treatment.

Plasma renin activity was reduced after one month of treatment and subsequently the values increased to control values.

Aldosterone did not show significant modifications. Plasma volume increased, but not significantly. No serious side effects were observed, nor were there any significant changes in haematological and biochemical variables.

Treatment of hypertensive patients with I.H.D. with alpha- and beta-adrenoreceptor blockade using Labetalol (600 mg/die) shows significant haemodynamic advantages compared with treatment by beta-receptor blockade alone.

Furthermore, treatment with Labetalol is useful in hypertensive patients with ischaemic heart disease.

The haemodynamic pattern of stable essential hypertension is characterized by normal or low cardiac output, and frequently by normal plasmatic volume while the systemic vascular resistances are always high [2, 5, 34].

The increase in S.V.R. could be a result of

an autoregulation phenomenon carried out by the organism to counterbalance the initial increase in cardiac output and plasma volume, determining tissue overperfusion [2, 7, 24, 34].

This increase in S.V.R. is a consequence also of structural changes in the precapillary resistance vessels with hyperactivity of smooth muscle cells of the vascular wall and exaggerated luminal reduction for a given vasoconstrictor stimulus [17].

Therefore, in the therapy of stable essential hypertension, the most important aim is to reduce the S.V.R. without changes in cardiac output and haematic perfusion of vital organs such as the brain and heart, especially when in the arterial wall there are atherosclerotic lesions.

In fact, the arterial hypertension treatment on the one hand diminishes the morbidity and mortality of cerebrovascular disease, but on the other hand does not influence the I.H.D. incidence [40-42]; this could happen because the decrease in tensive values sometimes determines a coronary flow reduction that can be prejudicial if, at the same time, there is not a decrease in the myocardial oxygen requirement as occurs when using the beta-adrenergic blocking drugs.

In fact, anti-hypertensive therapy using beta-adrenergic blocker drugs only sometimes has determined, a decrease in tensive values and a reduction in sudden death, myocardial infarction and reinfarction.

Labetalol has recently been approved for use in hypertension and represents the forerunner of a new pharmacological group of compounds with combined alpha- and beta-adrenoreceptor blocking properties [9, 13, 15, 23].

Like propranolol, Labetalol is unselective with respect to beta$_1$,- and beta$_2$-adrenoreceptors and is without sympathomimetic activity [8].

The ratio of the alpha- and beta-adrenoreceptor blocking effects is about 1:3 after oral administration [32].

It has been suggested that a combination of alpha- and beta-adrenoreceptor blocking drugs should be ideal for lowering the blood pressure since the latter should block the reflex effects of the former when the peripheral resistances are lowered by vasodilation [19].

During chronic treatment with Labetalol, 300 to 1200 gr for a few days and up to 16 months, there is a significant reduction in heart rate as well as in blood pressure [3, 20-21, 27].

The effect of Labetalol in decreasing peripheral resistances is in direct contrast to the effects of conventional beta-adrenoreceptor blocking drugs which cause an initial increase in peripheral resistances [39] and is compatible with its alpha-adrenoceptor blocking action.

In resting subjects with hypertension oral administration of Labetalol usually does not lower cardiac output [14, 21, 27].

In previous papers [28, 36] we have demonstrated that Labetalol administrated i.v. significantly lowers systolic, diastolic and effort blood pressure and improves the rest flow at the calf differently from the non-cardioselective beta-blocker drugs [28, 37].

Furthermore, it has been demonstrated that i.v. infusion of Labetalol increases the exercise tolerance of patients with angina pectoris [6, 11].

Labetalol, in fact, decreases the afterload, the heart rate and the pressure rate product both at rest and during exercise, thus limiting the external heart work load and the MVO_2 [12, 27, 36].

On the basis of these characteristics of Labetalol we thought it useful for the treatment of patients with essential hypertension and ischaemic heart disease. In particular we evaluated:

1. if Labetalol is suitable for enhancing the exertional angina threshold in hypertensive patients with stable effort angina pectoris;

2. if Labetalol was useful in relieving spontaneous chest pain episodes in two hypertensive patients with variant angina who partially benefited from short-term treatment with nifedipine 10 mg every 6 hours;

3. if the decrease in tensive values induced by Labetalol is maintained during chronic treatment;

4. the changes in systemic haemodynamics and in the haemodynamics in the peripheral district of the lower limbs during chronic administration of the drug;

5. the influence of chronic treatment with Labetalol on the renin-angiotensin-aldosterone system, on plasmatic volume, serum electrolytes and on biochemical variables.

Materials and methods:

6 males and 6 females aged 40 to 72 years, with an average age of 54 ± 11.5 years, were studied.

All patients were suffering from essential moderate-to-severe hypertension and ischaemic heart disease.

Ten hypertensive patients were also suffering from stable effort angina pectoris and two from both at rest and exertional angina.

All patients consented to participate in the study after being informed in detail of its nature and purpose.

A placebo was administered initially three times daily for 14 days to the patients with hypertension and stable angina pectoris; isosorbide dinitrate was given in case of need. Then oral Labetalol was administered, 200 mg t.i.d. for six months.

For three weeks, over alternating 48-hour periods, the two patients with hypertension and variant angina took either placebo four times a day or nifedipine 10 mg every 6 hours; then, Labetalol 200 mg t.i.d. and nifedipine 10 mg every 6 hours were given for six months.

During the placebo period and one, three and six months after beginning active treatment, the following parameters were evaluated:

1. effort chest pain episodes weekly in patients with stable angina pectoris;
2. spontaneous chest pain episodes weekly in patients with angina at rest;
3. angina threshold during bicycle ergometer test in both groups of patients;
4. systolic and diastolic blood pressure, heart rate, pressure rate product[2], ST-T segment depression, at rest and during exercise. These parameters were evaluated at the same work load achieved during treatment with placebo.

A graded, uninterrupted exercise test was started at 20 Watts for 3 minutes and the work load was increased by 20 W every 3 minutes until chest pain onset or exhaustion or blood pressure of 250/150 mmHg was reached; blood pressure, heart rate and E.C.G. in the V_4-V_5-V_6 leads were recorded at each minute during exercise and for 15 minutes in the recovery period.

5. Mean Blood Pressure (M.B.P. = S.B.P. + 2 D.B.P. / 3 = mmHg), Cardiac Output (C.O. = ml/min), obtained by the radiocardiographic method after i.v. administration of 50 microcuries of I^{131} labelled albumin, Stroke Volume (S.V. = C.O./H.R. = ml/beat), Systemic Vascular Resistances (S.V.R. = M.B.P. x 60 x 1332/C.O. = dynes/sec/cm^{-5}), Rest Flow (R.F. = ml/min/100 gr. muscle tissue) and Peak Flow (P.F. = ml/min/100 gr. muscle tissue, obtained after three minutes' arterial occlusion at 270 mmHg counterpressure), evaluated at the calf by strain-gauge plethysmography, Basal Vascular Resistances (B.V.R. = M.B.P.-/R.F.) and Minimal Vascular Resistances (M.V.R. = M.B.P./P.F.), arbitrarily obtained in the lower limbs district by means of the M.B.P./Arterial Flow ratio;

6. Plasma Renin Activity (P.R.A. = $\mu g/ml/h$) and Plasma Aldosterone ($\mu g/ml$) determined by radioimmunoassay, Plasma Volume (P.V. = ml/kg) obtained 10 minutes after i.v. administration of 5 microcuries of I^{131} labelled albumin, Serum Creatinine (mg per 100 ml of blood), Serum Electrolytes (mEq/1) and body weight.

Statistical analysis was performed using Student's t test for paired comparison. The dispersion of the data is mean $\pm$ standard deviation (S.D.)

Results:

Effort chest pain episodes:

Chronic treatment with Labetalol determined a significant decrease in chest pain episodes in patients with stable angina pectoris from 13 ± 9 with placebo to 6 ± 3 after one month of drug administration and to 5 ± 3 and 4 ± 2 after three and six months of therapy respectively (Table I).

Spontaneous chest pain episodes with ST-T segment elevation:

In two patients with variant angina nifedi-

Table I. *Effect of Labetalol in chest pain episodes and in work at the onset of exertional angina in patients with stable angina pectoris (mean ± S.D.).*

Parameters	Placebo	Chronic treatment with Labetalol 200 mg t.i.d.			p		
		after 1 month	after 3 months	after 6 months			
	1	2	3	4	1 → 2	1 → 3	1 → 4
EFFORT CHEST PAIN EPISODES	13 ± 9	6 ± 3	5 ± 3	4 ± 2	0.025	0.125	0.005
WORK LOAD AT ONSET ON ANGINA (kgm)	1254 ± 789	1942 ± 645	1984 ± 662	1990 ± 665	0.025	0.025	0.025

pine treatment reduced the chest pain episodes by half and then the nifedipine-labetalol association determined a further reduction (Table II).

Work load at the onset of exertional angina:

Labetalol administration induced a significant increase in the exertional angina threshold after one month of treatment as well as after three and six months of therapy (Table 1).

Blood pressure, pulse rate, pressure rate product^{-2} and ST-T segment depression at rest and during exercise:

Mean values and standard deviations of these parameters as measured before, as well as the changes observed after one, three and six months of treatment are given in Table III and in Figs. 1 and 2.

The pre-treatment average blood pressure was 198/112 mmHg at rest in the supine,

Table II. *Spontaneous chest pain episodes with ST-T segment weekly elevation in two patients with variant angina.*

	P	N	N + L after I month	N + L after 3 months	N + L after 6 months
GIUSEPPINA C.	17	8	5	3	I
BENITO S.	14	6	4	2	0

P = PLACEBO
N = NIFEDIPINE 10 mg every 6 hours
N + L = NIFEDIPINE 10 mg every 6 hours and LABETALOL 200 mg every 8 hours

188/119 mmHg in the upright position and 224/132 mmHg during exercise.

Chronic treatment with Labetalol determined a significant decrease in systolic (by 21 to 30 mmHg) and diastolic (by 15 to 18 mmHg) blood pressure under all conditions.

At rest, both in the supine and upright posture, diastolic blood pressure was affected more than systolic blood pressure.

A postural hypotension was not seen in any patient during the whole period of the study.

Heart rate was signifiantly reduced in all

conditions, at rest both in the supine (-8 beats per minute) and in the upright posture (-9 beats per minute) as well as during the bicycle ergometer test (-16 beats per minute).

The pressure rate product^{-2} was significantly affected both at rest (-20% after one month and -24% after six months of treatment) and during exercise (-21% and -22% respectively after one and six months of therapy).

Exercise-induced ST-T segment depression also diminished significantly.

Table III. *Effect of Labetalol on B.P., H.R., D.P.$^{-2}$, and $\downarrow$ ST at rest and during exercise (mean $\pm$ S.D.).*

Parameters		Placebo	Chronic treatment with Labetalol 200 mg t.i.d.			p		
			after 1 month	after 3 months	after 6 months			
		1	2	3	4	1 → 2	1 → 3	1 → 4
S.B.P. (mmHg)	supine	198.88 ± 15.36	176.66 ± 18.02	166.76 ± 17.01	168.87 ± 18.07	0.025	0.0005	0.0005
	upright	188.78 ± 16.35	168.33 ± 19.95	163.5 ± 15.07	164.2 ± 16.01	0.01	0.0025	0.0025
	exercise	224.7 ± 25.08	203.7 ± 21.07	199.5 ± 19.04	201 ± 20.02	0.025	0.01	0.025
D.B.P. (mmHg)	supine	112.44 ± 7.68	97.44 ± 10.13	95.72 ± 11.02	96.6 ± 10.5	0.025	0.025	0.0025
	upright	119.55 ± 7.81	103.15 ± 9.93	100.78 ± 9.78	101.27 ± 10.01	0.0005	0.0005	0.0005
	exercise	132.10 ± 15.01	117.1 ± 16.05	115.7 ± 15.02	116.8 ± 15.72	0.025	0.025	0.025
H.R. (b/min)	supine	80.5 ± 8.78	71.9 ± 7.15	72.1 ± 7.02	71.7 ± 7.27	0.025	0.025	0.0125
	upright	85.7 ± 11.02	77.4 ± 8.04	76.02 ± 7.88	76.55 ± 7.98	0.05	0.025	0.025
	exercise	119.2 ± 17.02	102.7 ± 13.04	104.8 ± 13.75	103.22 ± 12.75	0.025	0.025	0.025
D.P.$^{-2}$	at rest	160.09 ± 13.48	127.01 ± 12.88	120.23 ± 11.01	121.07 ± 11.07	0.0005	0.0005	0.0005
	exercise	267.39 ± 32.68	209.19 ± 25.47	209.07 ± 24.78	207.47 ± 23.07	0.0005	0.0005	0.0005
ST (mm)$^{-2}$	at rest	0.85 ± 0.85	0.45 ± 0.4	0.48 ± 0.45	0.4 ± 0.37	N.S.	N.S.	N.S.
	exercise	2.38 ± 0.97	1.32 ± 0.78	1.35 ± 0.88	1.42 ± 0.79	0.0125	0.0125	0.025

Systemic haemodynamics

Mean blood pressure decreased significantly from 141.94 ± 10.44 mmHg to 124.34 ± 12.51 mmHg after one month of treatment with Labetalol and to 120.54 ± 12.28 and 121.46 ± 12.51 mmHg after three and six months respectively.

Cardiac output did not show any change because an increase in stroke volume (significant after one month of therapy only) entirely counterbalanced the heart rate reduction.

Systemic vascular resistances significantly decreased from 1949 ± 174.49 dynes/sec/cm.$^{-5}$ during the placebo period, to 1672.93 ± 165.02 after one month and to 1649.58 ± 161.07 after three months of treatment: a slight increase was observed after six months to 1752.18 ± 179.17 dynes/sec/cm^{-5}.

Peripheral haemodynamics in the lower limbs district (Table V and Fig. 4):

Rest flow at the calf increased significantly after chronic treatment with Labetalol, while peak flow did not show important changes. Both basal and minimal resistances decreased significantly, but B.V.R. fell more than M.V.R.

Plasma volume (Table VI):

Long-term therapy with Labetalol induced a slight but non-significant increase in plasma volume, more evident after three and six months of drug administration.

Plasma renin activity and aldosterone (Table VI):

P.R.A. was significantly reduced after one month of treatment returning then to control levels, while plasmatic aldosterone did not show any changes.

Biochemical variables and body weight (Table VI):

No significant changes were observed.

Discussion:

Treatment with Labetalol, 200 mg t.i.d., for six months has determined a significative improvement in subjective symptomatology and an important reduction in tensive values in hypertensive patients with ischaemic heart disease.

89

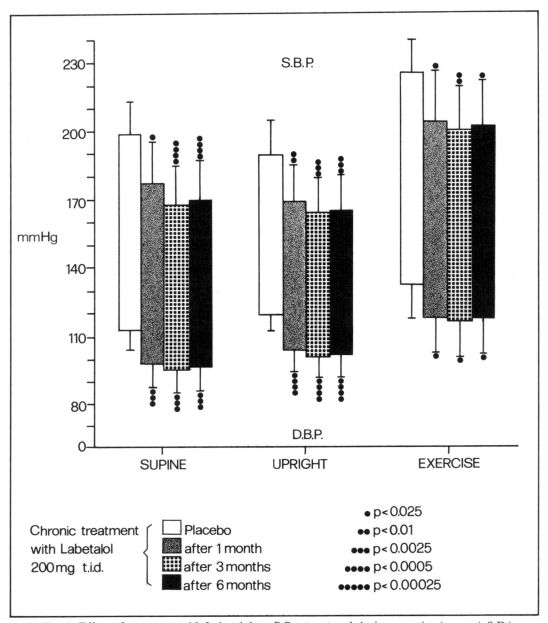

Fig. 1. Effect of treatment with Labetalol on B.P. at rest and during exercise (mean ± S.D.).

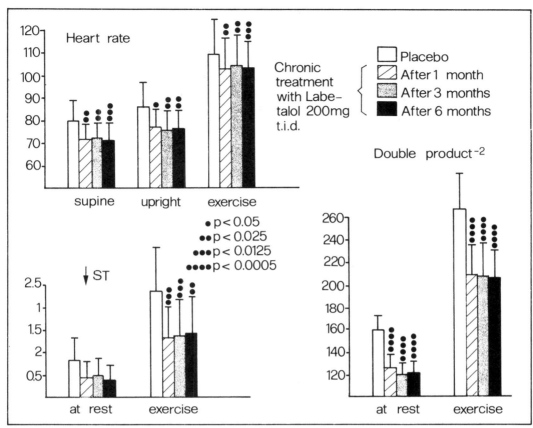

Fig. 2. Effect of treatment with Labetalol on H.R. ↓ST and D.P.$^{-2}$ at rest and during exercise (mean ± S.D.).

Table IV. *Effect of Labetalol on M.B.P. and systemic haemodynamics (mean ± S.D.).*

Parameters	Placebo	Chronic treatment with Labetalol 200 mg t.i.d.			p		
		after 1 month	after 3 months	after 6 months			
	1	2	3	4	1 → 2	1 → 3	1 → 4
M.B.P. (mmHg)	141.94 ± 10.44	124.34 ± 12.51	120.54 ± 12.28	121.46 ± 12.51	0.0025	0.0005	0.0005
H.R. upright (b/min)	85.7 ± 11.02	77.4 ± 8.04	76.02 ± 7.88	76.55 ± 7.99	0.025	0.025	0.025
C.O. (b/min)	5.82 ± 1.12	5.94 ± 0.57	5.84 ± 0.66	5.84 ± 0.93	N.S.	N.S.	N.S.
S.V. (ml/b)	70.03 ± 11.31	79.57 ± 7.50	78.85 ± 8.85	74.74 ± 12.20	0.025	N.S.	N.S.
S.V.R. (dynes sec cm^{-5})	1949 ± 174.49	1672.93±165.02	1649.58±161.07	1752.18±179.17	0.0025	0.0025	0.0025

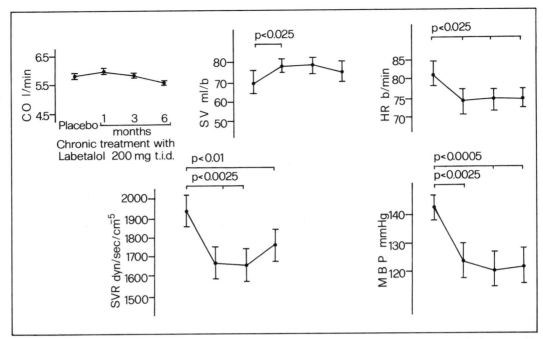

Fig. 3. Effect of treatment with Labetalol on M.B.P. and systemic haemodynamics at rest and during exercise (mean ± S.D.).

Table V. *Effect of Labetalol on peripheral haemodynamics in the lower limbs districts (mean ± S.D.).*

Parameters	Placebo	Chronic treatment with Labetalol 200 mg t.i.d.			p		
		after 1 month	after 3 months	after 6 months			
	1	2	3	4	1 → 2	1 → 3	1 → 4
R.F. ml/min/100 gr muscle tissue	3.66 ± 2.08	5.64 ± 2.30	5.09 ± 1.84	5.01 ± 1.97	0.05	0.01	0.05
P.F. ml/min/100 gr muscle tissue	21.54 ± 7.95	23.54 ± 7.27	23.10 ± 6.88	21.07 ± 7.75	N.S.	N.S.	N.S.
B.V.R. (A.U.)	38.78 ± 10.51	22.04 ± 5.07	23.68 ± 4.66	24.24 ± 5.97	0.0005	0.0005	0.0005
M.V.R. (A.U.)	6.58 ± 1.1	5.28 ± 1.07	5.21 ± 1.21	5.76 ± 1.27	0.005	0.005	0.005

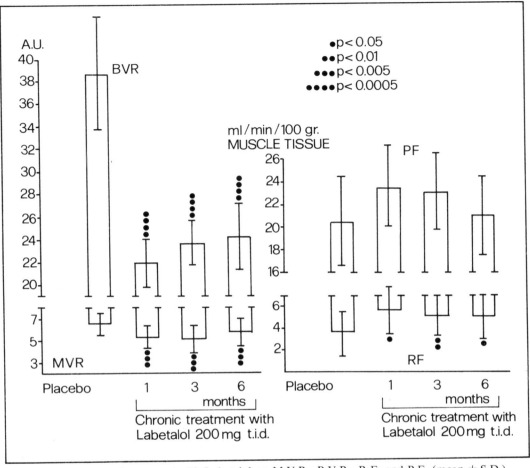

Fig. 4. Effect of treatment with Labetalol on M.V.R., B.V.R., R.F. and P.F. (mean ± S.D.).

The reduction in effort chest pain episodes and the increase in the work load threshold for exertional angina are consequences of the diminution of external heart work and myocardial MVO_2 induced by Labetalol.

That agrees with our previous findings [29, 36] obtained in hypertensive patients after i.v. infusion of Labetalol (1 mg/kg body weight) and according to reports by Metha [27] and Cherchi [12] which demonstrated a reduction in pressure rate product and in pressure rate ejection time product respectively in hypertensive patients and in patients with I.H.D.; Boakes also reported that Labetalol increased acute exercise tolerance in patients with effort angina.

Our study demonstrates that improved exercise tolerance, in patients with angina pectoris, persists after chronic treatment also.

There is no experience in the management of variant angina perctoris with Labetalol. But alpha-adrenoreceptor-mediated coronary spasm is now recognized as a possible cause of angina pectoris, especially variant angina [26]; thus, calcium inhibitors are extremely useful for these indications [26], but Labetalol with its alpha-adrenergic blocking properties might prove just as useful as calcium antagonists in this affection. In our experience the nifedipine-labetalol association significantly prevents spontaneous chest pain episodes perhaps because the alpha-adrenoreceptor blockade induced by La-

Table VI. *Effect of Labetalol on P.V., P.R.A., Aldosterone, biochemical variables, and body weight (mean ± S.D.).*

| Parameters | Placebo | Chronic treatment with Labetalol 200 mg t.i.d. | | | p | | |
| | | after 1 month | after 3 months | after 6 months | | | |
	1	2	3	4	1 → 2	1 → 3	1 → 4
P.V. (ml/kg)	43.95 ± 8.636	44.781 ± 7.36	48.109 ± 6.06	47.92 ± 5.31	N.S.	N.S.	N.S.
P.R.A. (ng/ml/h)	2.15 ± 1.25	1.28 ± 0.78	1.62 ± 0.84	1.68 ± 0.90	0.05	N.S.	N.S.
ALDOSTERONE (pg/ml)	217.5 ± 79.47	193.75 ± 34.97	213.75 ± 104.51	225 ± 129.03	N.S.	N.S.	N.S.
CREATININE (mg%)	1.2 ± 0.25	1.25 ± 0.32	1.21 ± 0.27	1.19 ± 0.28	N.S.	N.S.	N.S.
B.U.N. (gr%)	0.45 ± 0.09	0.47 ± 0.08	0.46 ± 0.09	0.46 ± 0.085	N.S.	N.S.	N.S.
SODIUM (mEq/l)	141 ± 2.75	140 ± 19	140.5 ± 2	141 ± 1.7	N.S.	N.S.	N.S.
POTASSIUM (mEq/l)	4.4 ± 0.35	4.42 ± 0.37	4.37 ± 0.45	4.39 ± 0.51	N.S.	N.S.	N.S.
CHLORIDEMIA (mEq/l)	140.2 ± 2.89	103.87 ± 2.75	103.72 ± 2.88	104.1 ± 2.8	N.S.	N.S.	N.S.
BODY WEIGHT (ml/kg)	71.1 ± 6.89	72.21 ± 7.02	72.2 ± 6.85	7.21 ± 7.84	N.S.	N.S.	N.S.

betalol can strengthen the spasmolytic properties of nifedipine. Therefore, these findings need confirmation in larger series of patients.

In contrast with beta-adrenergic blocking drugs, Labetalol reduces blood pressure without lowering cardiac output and decreases the systemic vascular resistances, too.

This drug, which combines the properties of blocking both the alpha-adrenoreceptors of the resistance vessels and the beta-adrenoreceptors in the heart, diminishes blood pressure by decreasing the peripheral resistances and, at the same time inhibits the reflex increase in heart rate and cardiac output.

Thus, Labetalol decreases blood pressure without modifying the tissue perfusion.

The haemodynamic changes found in our study agree with those obtained by Koch [21], after chronic treatment but partially differ from those of Fagard and coworkers who after 2.44 weeks of treatment observed a decrease both in S.V.R. and C.O. [16].

This difference should be a result of the higher dose used by these authors (1650 mg daily).

In our study we have also evaluated the haemodynamics in the peripheral district of the lower limbs. Labetalol, according to its alpha-blocking properties, reduces the vascular resistances at the calf both in basal conditions and after ischaemic stimulus, increasing also the rest flow evaluated by strain-gauge plethysmography.

Thus, the long-term oral as well as i.v. infusion [28, 37], or acute oral [29] administration of Labetalol does not reduce the tissue perfusion at the calf like non-cardioselective beta-adrenergic blocking drugs; therefore, Labetalol can also be useful in hypertensive patients with intermittent claudication.

Oral Labetalol, 600 mg daily, given for six months produced no significative changes in plasma renin activity [9, 27].

Our experience agrees with these findings but contrasts with Koch's report [21].

This difference may be a consequence of the

different dosages employed. In fact, in his study [21] the patients took 1200 mg daily of Labetalol; it is possible that such a dosage inhibits the renin secretion while at lower dosages the inhibition of renin release mediated by the beta-adrenoreceptor blockade could be counterbalanced by renin release stimulation mediated by the alpha-adrenoreceptor blockade [10, 35].

In our study chronic treatment with Labetalol slightly increases the plasmatic volume; it could be interesting to evaluate the behaviour of this parameter in longer treatment because the expansion of plasmatic volume could be a limiting mechanism of the anti-hypertensive action.

However, the expansion of volume can be completely avoided by discontinuous administration of diuretic drugs.

The complete lack of side effects of the drug after six months of treatment is noteworthy.

In conclusion, Labetalol is a useful drug in the treatment of hypertensive patients with ischaemic heart disease. In fact, the drug significantly reduces blood pressure both at rest, in the supine and upright posture and during exercise, increases the work load threshold for exertional angina and improves the subjective symptomatology preventing exertional angina and spontaneous chest pain episodes in patients with angina pectoris.

The haemodynamic changes induced by Labetalol are such that the drug does not reduce but improves tissue perfusion (at least in the peripheral district of the lower limbs that we have studied).

References

1. Ahlmark G., Saetre H., Korsgren M.: Letter: Reduction of sudden deaths after myocardial infarction. *Lancet*, 2, 1563, 1974.
2. Allen W.C.: The concept of autoregulation of total blood flow and its role in hypertension. *Am. J. Med.*, 68, 906, 1980.
3. Andersson O., Berglund G., Hansson L.: Antihypertensive action, time of onset and effects on carbohydrate metabolism of labetalol. *Brit. J. Clin. Pharmacol.*, 3, Suppl., 757, 1976.
4. Berglund G., Wilhelmsen L., Sammerstedt R., Hansson L., Andersson O., Silversston R., Wedel H., Wikstrand J.: Coronary heart disease after treatment of hypertension. *Lancet*, 1, I, 1978.
5. Birkenhager W.H., Schalekamp A.D.H., Krauss X.H., Kolsters G., Schalekamp-Kujken M.P.A., Kroon B.J.M., Teulings F.A.G.: Systemic and renal haemodynamics, body fluid and renin in benign essential hypertension with special reference to natural history. *Eur. J. Clin. Invest.* 2, 115, 1972.
6. Boakes A.J., Prichard B.N.C.: The effect of AH 5158, pindolol, propranolol and D-propranolol on acute exercise tolerance in angina pectoris. *Br. J. Pharmacol.*, 47, 673, 1973.
7. Borst J.G.G., Borst de Gens A.: Hypertension explained by Starling's theory of circulatory homeostasis. *Lancet*, 1, 677, 1963.
8. Brittain R.T., Levy G.P.: A review of the animal pharmacology of labetalol, a combined alpha- and beta-adrenoreceptor blocking drug. *Brit. J. Clin. Pharmacol.*, 3, Suppl. 3, 681, 1976.
9. Brodgen R.N., Heel R.C., Speight T.M., Avery G.S.: Labetalol: a review of its pharmacology and therapeutic use in hypertension. *Drugs*, 15, 4, 251, 1978.
10. Chapman B.P.: Labetalol and urinary catecholamines. *Brit. Med. J.*, I, 6109, 364, 1978.
11. Cherchi A., Fonzo R., Lai C., Mercuro G.: Influenza del labetalolo sul test di tolleranza allo sforzo in pazienti affetti da angina pectoris. pp. 40-54. In: *Atti Conv. Int. Ipertensione: Nuove prospettive terapeutiche.* Venezia, 18-20 maggio 1978. Glaxo Italia 1978, 269.
12. Cherchi A., Raffo M., Sau F., Pirisi R., Seguro C.: Sull'influenza della terapia antiipertensiva mediante labetalolo e clortalidone sul doppio e triplo prodotto a riposo e sotto sforzo. *Atti del Congresso Nazionale Società Italiana Cardiologia*, Florence, 1980.
13. Collier J.G., Dawnay N.A.H., Nachev C.H., Robinson B.F.: Clinical investigation of an antagonist at alpha- and beta-adrenoreceptors: AH 5158 A. *Brit. J. Pharmacol.*, 44, 286, 1972.
14. Edward R.C., Raftery E.B.: Haemodynamic effects of long-term oral labetalol. *Brit. J. Clin. Pharmacol.* 3, Suppl., 733, 1976.
15. Farmer J.B., Kennedy I., Levy G.P., Marshall R.J.: Pharmacology of AH 5158; a drug which blocks alpha and beta-adrenoceptors. *Brit. J. Pharmacol.*, 45, 660, 1972.
16. Fagard R., Amery A., Reybrouck T., Lijnen P., Billiet L.: Response of the systemic and pulmonary circulation to alpha- and beta-receptor blockade (Labetalol) at rest and during exercise in hypertensive patients. *Circulation*, 60, 6, 1214, 1979.
17. Folkow B.: Vascular changes in hypertension: review and recent animal studies. In: (Eds.) G. Berglund, L. Hansson and L. Werko. *Pathophysiology and management of arterial hypertension*, p.95, Mollodal, Sweden, Lindgren and Soner, 1975.
18. Frishman W., Halprin S.: Clinical pharmacology of the new beta-adrenergic blocking drugs. Part 7. New horizons in beta-adrenoceptor blockade therapy: Labetalol. *Am. Heart J.*, 98, 5, 660, 1979.
19. Gilmore E., Weil J., Chidsey C.: Treatment of essential hypertension with a new vasodilator in combina-

tion with beta-adrenergic blockade. *New Engl. J. Med.*, 282, 521, 1970.

20. Koch G.: Combined alpha- and beta-adrenoceptor blockade with oral labetalol in hypertensive patients with reference to haemodynamic effects at rest and during exercise. *Brit. J. Clin. Pharmacol.*, 3, Suppl. 729, 1976.

21. Koch G.: Haemodynamic adaptation at rest and during exercise to long-term antihypertensive treatment with combined alpha- and beta-adrenoceptor blockade by labetalol. *Br. Heart. J.*, 41, 192, 1979.

22. Koch-Weiser J.: Vasodilator drugs in the treatment of hypertension. *Arch. Intern. Med.*, 133, 1017, 1974.

23. Hansson L., Hanel B.: Labetalol, a new alpha- and beta-blocking agent in hypertension. *Brit. J. Clin. Pharmacol.* 3, Suppl., 763, 1976.

24. Ledingham J.M., Cohen R.D.: Autoregulation of the total systemic circulation and its relation to control of cardiac output and arterial pressure. *Lancet*, 1, 887, 1963.

25. Majid P.A., Meeran, M.K., Benaim M.E., Sharma B., Taylor S.H.: Alpha- and beta-adrenergic receptor blockade in the treatment of hypertension. *Br. Heart J.*, 36, 588, 1974.

26. Maseri A., L'Abbate A, Baroldi G., Chierchia S., Marzilli M., Ballestra A.M., Severi S., Parodi O., Biagini A., Distante A., Pesola A.: Coronary vasospasm as a possible cause of myocardial infarction. *New Engl. J. Med.*, 299, 1271, 1978.

27. Metha J., Cohn J.N.: Haemodynamic effects of labetalol, an alpha- and beta-adrenergic blocking agent in hypertensive subjects. *Circulation*, 55, 370, 1977.

28. Novo S., Pinto A., Davì G., Riolo F., Gullotti D.: Su alcuni effetti cardiovascolari della somministrazione acuta di labetalolo in soggetti ipertesi. *Boll. Soc. Ital. Cardiol.* 25, 2, 149, 1980.

29. Novo S., Pinto A., Davì G., La Menza B., Strano A.: Effects of beta-blocking adrenergic drugs on arterial flow of the lower limbs. *Proceedings of XII World Congress of Angiology*, Athens, September 6-12, 1980.

30. Olivari M.T., Bartorelli C., Polese A., Fiorentini C., Moruzzi P., Guazzi M.: Treatment of hypertension with nifedipine, a calcium antagonist agent. *Circulation*, 59, 5, 1979.

31. Page L.B., Yager H.M., Sidd J.J.: Drugs in the management of hypertension. Part III. *Am. Heart J.*, 92, 252, 1976.

32. Richards D.A., Tuckman J., and Prichard B.N.C.: Combined alpha- and beta-adrenoceptor blockade with labetalol at rest and during exercise. *Brit. J. Clin. Pharmacol.*, 3, 967, 1976.

33. Richards D.A., Pricard B.N.C.: Circulatory and alpha-adrenoceptor blocking effects of phentolamine. *Brit. J. Clin. Pharmacol.*, 5, 507, 1978.

34. Safar M.E., Chau N.P., Weiss Y.A., London G.M., Simon A.C.H., Milliez P.P.: The pressure-volume relationship in normotensive and permanent essential hypertensive patients. *Clin. Sci. Mol. Med.*, 50, 207, 1976.

35. Salvetti A., Pedrinelli R., Cavasini L, Lera M., Poli L., Sassano P.: L'effetto di dosi crescenti di labetalolo sul sistema renina-angiotensina-aldosterone e sulla pressione arteriosa di pazienti con ipertensione essentiale. pp. 128-140. In: *Atti Conv. Int. Ipertensione: Nuove prospettive terapeutiche.* Venezia, 18-20 maggio 1978. Glaxo Italia 1978, 269.

36. Strano A., Novo S., Davì G., Pinto A., Riolo F.: Comportamento dei valori tensivi arteriosi e della reattività vascolare a riposo e dopo sforzo in soggetti ipertesi trattati con labetalolo per via endovenosa. pp. 93-102. In *Atti Conv. Int. Ipertensione: Nuove prospettive terapeutiche.* Venezia, 18-20 maggio 1978. Glaxo Italia 1978, 269.

37. Strano A., Novo S., Pinto A., Davì G.: The effects of beta-blocking agents on the arterial flow of the lower limbs using strain-gauge plethysmography. *Proceedings of Ist International Colloquy of Angiology*, Florence, October 23-26, 1979.

38. Strano A., Novo S., Licata G., Salerno L., Pinto A., Davì G., Botindari G.: Nifedipine-acebutolol association in arterial hypertension. *Atti del II° Simposio Mediterraneo su Nuovi Aspetti Terapeutici nell'angina pectoris e nell'ipertensione.*

39. Tarazi R.D., Duston H.P.: Beta-adrenergic blockade in hypertension. Practical and theoretical implications of long-term haemodynamic variations. *Am. J. Cardiol.*, 29, 633, 1972.

40. Veterans Administration Study on Antihypertensive Agents. *J.A.M.A.*, 202, 1028, 1967.

41. Veterans Administration Study on Antihypertensive Agents. *J.A.M.A.*, 213, 1143, 1970.

42. Veterans Administration Study on Antihypertensive Agents. *Circulation*, 45, 991, 1972.

Hypertension, recent advances and research
edited by M. Condorelli, A. Zanchetti
Cortina International, Verona 1982

Adrenergic receptors and myocardial ischaemia

M. CHIARIELLO, G. BREVETTI, A. GENOVESE

Institute of Medical Pathology, 2nd School of Medicine, Naples, Italy

Key words. Adrenergic Receptors; Myocardial Ischaemia; Coronary Steal; Vasodilating Agents; Vasocontriction; Regional Myocardial Blood Flow; Methoxamine; Myocardial Creatinkinase; Infarct Size; Reverse Coronary Steal.

Summary. The phenomenon of "coronary steal", i.e., the shunting of blood from ischaemic to normally perfused areas of the myocardium, has been described as an effect of the administration of several vasodilating agents. This study was performed to ascertain whether the reverse situation can be induced, i.e. whether vasoconstriction of the vessels supplying the non-ischaemic zone could increase the collateral flow to the ischaemic area. In 16 open-chest dogs, 15 and 30 min. after occlusion of the left anterior descending coronary artery, epicardial electrograms were recorded and regional myocardial blood flow (RMBF) was measured with radiolabeled microspheres. Methoxamine was infused intravenously between 17 and 30 min. the mean arterial pressure being kept constant. The results indicate that while the coronary arterial flow to the normal myocardium fell from 90.6 ± 4.3 to 77.7 ± 3.2 ml/min/100 g (P < 0.01), the collateral blood flow to the ischaemic area increased from 21.4 ± 3.5 to 41.0 ± 4.2 ml/min/100 g (P < 0.01), and thereby reduced acute myocardial ischaemic injury. This favourable redistribution of blood flow might be considered a "reverse coronary steal".

The local or systemic release of catecholamines induced by stress has been considered for many years an important factor in attacks of angina pectoris and in the development of myocardial infarction. Actually, stress reaction may produce sympathetic overactivity, with release of catecholamines, increase in heart rate and in myocardial contractility and a consequent increase in oxygen consumption. This will result in a worsening of the temporary imbalance between oxygen supply and demand and, therefore, in an aggravation of the acute myocardial ischaemia. It seems, therefore, relevant to believe that sympathetic overactivity and release of catecholamines could play an important rôle in the infarction process. Several experimental studies seem to confirm this hypothesis: in the first place, isoproterenol infarctions are commonly used as a means of inducing myocardial necrosis [1-3].

Moreover, myocardial cell damage has been produced by perfusing isolated working rat hearts with norepinephrine in a concentration comparable to that obtainable in the myocardial tissue, if all of the stored epinephrine is released from the myocardial sympathetic nerve endings simultaneously [4]. Myocardial ischaemic damage was also produced by perfusing the isolated rat hearts with tyramine, which exerts its sympathetic action exclusively through the local release of stored endogenous norepinephrine [4].

Myocardial enzymatic and morphological changes induced by tyramine-released catecholamines have also been observed in the intact animal. Serial injections of increasing amounts of tyramine produced myocardial cell damage in rats as documented by the increase in serum creatinkinase isoenzyme MB-CK found 2 and 4 hours post-injection (Figs. 1, 2) as well as by

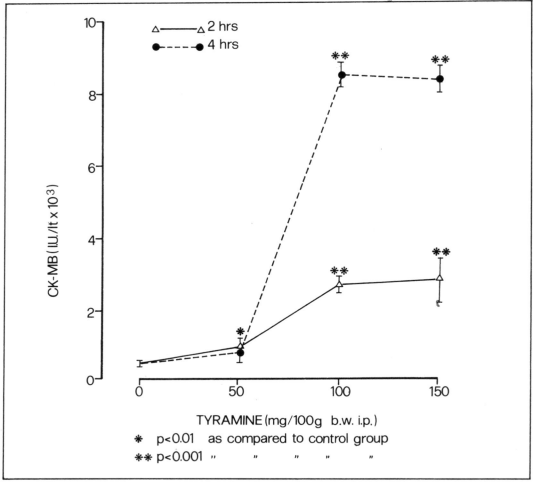

Fig. 1. Serum creatinkinase isoenzyme (MB-CK) levels (IU/L ± SEM) in Sprague-Dawley male rats treated i.p. with progressive doses of tyramine chlorhydrate (50, 100 and 150 mg/100 g body weight). MB-CK changes are evaluated 2 solid line) or 4 (broken line) hours after tyramine injection.

the depletion in CK activity in the homogenetes of whole myocardial tissue (Figs. 3, 4) [5]. The peak action of tyramine was observed 4 hours after the administration of the drug, as shown by the highest level of MB-CK serum concentration (Fig. 2) and the lowest myocardial CK activity found at that time (Fig. 4). Electron microscopic observations confirmed that tyramine-induced catecholamines were able to produce ischaemic myocardial damage (Figs. 5, 6).

Since catecholamines and sympathetic over-

activity appear to be harmful to the ischaemic myocardium, it has been suggested that beta-adrenoceptor blockade may be protective. Therefore, beta-blockers have been thoroughly studied to establish whether they were able to reduce myocardial damage following coronary artery occlusion by favourably altering the balance between myocardial oxygen requirements and delivery. Actually, a large number of studies have proved that beta-blockers are effective in reducing the electrocardiographic and enzymatic signs of myocardial injury and the

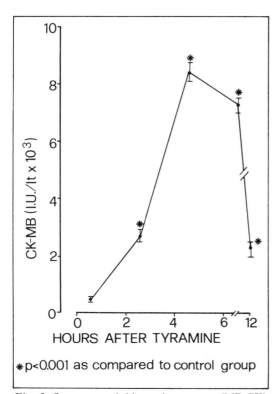

CK-MB (IU./lt x 10³)

HOURS AFTER TYRAMINE

*p<0.001 as compared to control group

Fig. 2. Serum creatinkinase isoenzyme (MB-CK) levels (IU/L ± SEM) evaluated in Sprague-Dawley male rats at different times (2, 4, 6, or 12 hours) after i.p. injection of tyramine chlorhydrate (100 mg/100 g body weight).

extent of myocardial necrosis in dogs [6, 7] and in preventing or reducing the ultrastructural changes induced by ischaemia in the rat myocardium [8]. Moreover, in human beings with acute anterior myocardial infarction the intravenous injection of propranolol was followed by a marked decrease in chest pain and ventricular irritability. The ST segment elevations in these patients fell strikingly, indicating that propranolol may reduce myocardial ischaemic injury and its manifestations. The exact mechanism by which beta-blockers decrease myocardial infarct size is not known; however, several hypotheses, which are not necessarily mutually exclusive, have been suggested.

The most widely accepted view is that beta-blockers act by reducing myocardial oxygen demands through their negative inotropic and chronotropic effects. It has also been proposed that beta-blocking drugs alter substrate utilization by the heart. In fact, it has been shown that propranolol, by blocking beta-adrenergic receptors decreases lipolysis and myocardial free fatty acid uptake and shifts the utilization of myocardial substrates to glucose during experimental myocardial infarction [9]. Thus, in patients with acute myocardial infarction, propranolol has been shown to shift the metabolism of the myocardium from free fatty acids to carbohydrates and to decrease myocardial oxygen consumption, while lactate reverts from production to extraction [10]. Finally, it has also been suggested that propranolol protects the ischaemic myocardium by exerting a primary protective effect on the microvasculature [11].

To decrease myocardial necrosis in acutely ischaemic hearts a reduction in oxygen consumption has also been sought through a reduction in afterload by the use of vasodilating drugs. Ganglionic or alpha-receptor blocking agents were used for this purpose and proved to be effective in reducing ischaemic injury and in amelioraing cardiac performance [12]. However, the practical use of these alpha-receptor blocking drugs in acute myocardial infarction has been limited by undesirable side effects, particularly on perfusion pressure.

Since both beta-adrenergic blocking agents, and interventions that decrease afterload reduce myocardial damage, it seemed reasonable that a drug possessing both these actions could be very effective in reducing infarct size. Therefore, the protective effects of Labetalol, a drug (with a proven ability to block effectively both beta₁- and beta₂-receptors and also possessing alpha-adrenergic blocking properties as well [13, 14], were assayed in experimental myocardial infarction induced in the rat by coronary artery occlusion [15]. This techinique enjoys the obvious advantages of allowing the quantity of necrotic left ventricular myocardium to be measured directly, both at the time of peak necrosis and on completion of the healing process.

The first method used was enzymatic and consisted in the measurement of the total creatinkinase activity remaining in the left ventricle

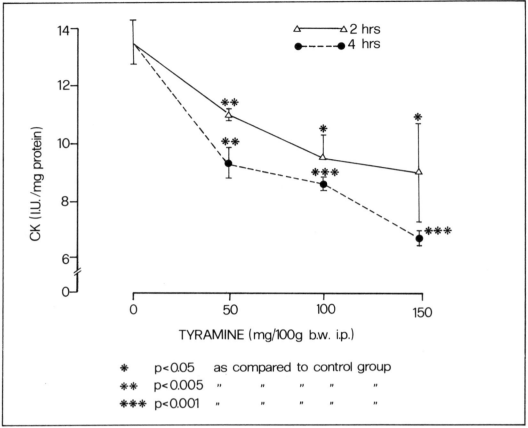

Fig. 3. Myocardial creatinkinase (CK) activity changes (IU/mg protein ± SEM) in Sprague-Dawley male rats treated i.p. with progressive doses of tiramine chlorhydrate. CK changes are evaluated 2 (solid line) or 4 (brochen line) hours after tyramine injection.

of rats 48 hours after coronary artery occlusion. From this value, the percent of infarcted left ventricular mass was calculated as previously reported [16]. By this method, the efficacy of Labetalol was evaluated and compared with that of propranolol given at a dose having comparable beta-blocking activity.

The results of these experiments indicate that Labetalol and propranolol are each effective in protecting the myocardium from ischaemic necrosis, but that the simultaneous blockade of alpha- and beta-receptors achieved by Labetalol appears more affective than the use of beta-receptor blockade alone (Fig. 7). These data can be explained by the further reduction in myocardial oxygen consumption due to the decrease in peripheral resistance induced by

alpha-adrenergic receptor blockade. The effects of Labetalol have also been exploited by quantitative histology: histological sections were prepared from rat hearts with myocardial infarctions produced by coronary occlusion performed either 48 hours or 21 days earlier and the infarcted area was measured by planimetry and expressed as a percent of the whole left ventricular area (Fig. 8).

By this method, which allows us to quantify directly the extent of experimental myocardial infarction both at the time of peak necrosis and on completion of scar formation, Labetalol proved to be extremely effective in reducing expected infarct size (Fig. 9). Thus, the simultaneous blockade of alpha- and beta-adrenoceptors permanently reduces infarct size

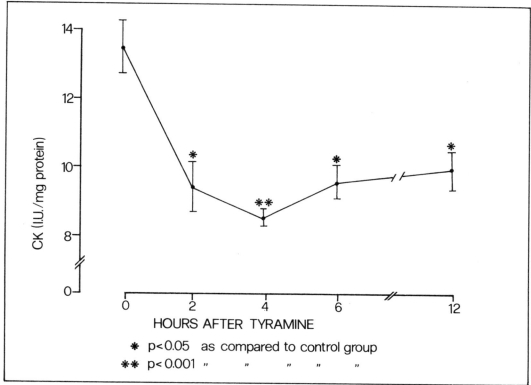

Fig. 4. Myocardial creatinkinase (CK) activity changes (IU/mg protein ± SEM) in Sprague-Dawley male rats at different times (2, 4, 6, or 12 hours) after i.p. injection of tyramine chlorhydrate (100 mg/100 g body weight).

in rats with coronary artery occlusion and its beneficial effects are greater than those of propranolol. These experimental data may open up new perspectives in the future treatment of ischaemic heart disease, in particular when treating patients with acute myocardial infarction. Although alpha-adrenergic blocking drugs under certain conditions and when associated with simultaneous beta-adrenergic blockade may prove beneficial to the ischaemic myocardium, through a reduction in cardiac work and thus in myocardial oxygen consumption, the opposite situation may occur when the drug-induced vasodilation favours the so-called "coronary steal" phenomenon. This event can take place whenever a sudden reduction in the vascular resistance of a given area results in the shunting of blood to it through collateral vessels from adjacent areas of unchanged resistance.

Coronary vasodilators given to patients with ishcaemic heart disease may increase the total coronary blood flow, but they may do this at the expense of reducing the collateral flow to the ischaemic zones already maximally dilated as a result of metabolic stimuli [17-22]. Since drugs which cause arterial dilation in the normal myocardium also reduce the arterial flow to ischaemic areas, it is been investigated whether interventions which cause arterial constriction in the normal myocardium, such as some alpha-receptor stimulating drugs, would increase the flow to the ischaemic areas, thus producing a "reverse coronary steal" [23]. In this study, in dogs with coronary artery occlusion, methoxamine was infused while systemic blood pressure was kept constant by bleeding. This infusion resulted in an increase in systemic as well as coronary artery resistance (Fig. 10).

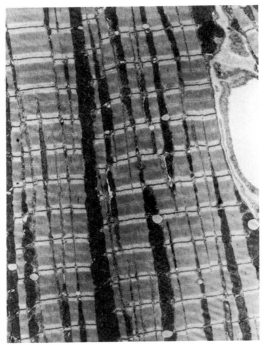

Fig. 5. Portion of myocardial fiber from control animal. The mitochondria are compact and have regularly distributed cristae. The Z bands are uniformly spaced and separated from the A bands by pale I bands containing myofibers. Glycogen is present in the form ot punctate dense granules. Lead hydroxide (x 11,200).

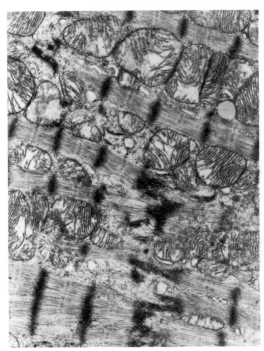

Fig. 6. Portion of myocardial fiber 4 hours after administration of i.p. tyramine (100 mg/100 g body weight). There is mitochondrial damage including swelling and destruction of cristae. Lead hydroxide (x 12,000).

As a consequence of the methoxamine-induced vasoconstriction, blood flow to the normal non-ischaemic myocardium decreased (Figs. 11, 12). However, collateral blood flow to the ischaemic sites rose significantly (Figs. 11, 13). Simultaneously with the increase in blood supply, also the electrocardiographic evidence of myocardial injury decreased, as shown by the fall in average ST segment elevation on the epicardial map (Fig. 14). The schematic representation of the hypothesis of reverse coronary steal is reported in Fig. 15. It is shown how the increase in coronary resistance in the normal myocardium induces a fall in flow to the non-ischaemic tissue, while the blood supply to the ischaemic zones through collateral vessels increases. The demonstration of the feasibility of producing a

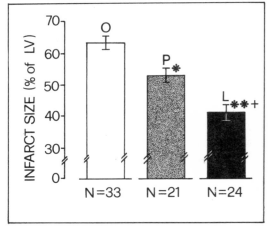

Fig. 7. Infarct size expressed as percent of left ventricle (LV) calculated by the creatinkinase method in 33 control (0), 21 propranolol-treated (P) and 24 Labetalol-treated rats (L), 48 hours after coronary artery occlusion. [* difference from control group, $p < 0.05$; ** = difference from control group, $p < 0.01$; + = difference from propranolol-treated group, $p < 0.05$].

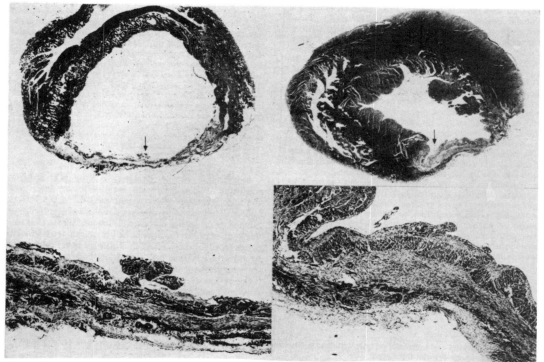

Fig. 8. Histological sections of transverse slices of rats killed 21 days after occlusion of the left main coronary artery. Left, the heart from a control rat at (top) low magnification (x 7.5) and (bottom) high magnification (x 42). Right, the heart from a Labetalol-treated rat at (top) low magnification (x 7.5) and (bottom) high magnification (x 42).

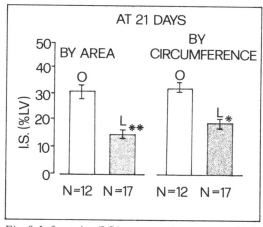

Fig. 9. Infarct size (I.S.) expressed as percent of left ventricle (LV) assessed on histological sections either by area or by the circumference method, 21 days after occlusion in control (0), and in Labetalol-treated (L) rats. [* = difference from control group, $p < 0.05$; ** = difference from control group, $p < 0.01$].

reverse coronary steal phenomenon does suggest that this principle may provide a useful approach to the treatment of different forms of regional myocardial ischaemia. In fact, by inducing a reverse coronary steal it may be possible to increase collateral flow to underperfused zones of the myocardium in patients with regional ischaemia.

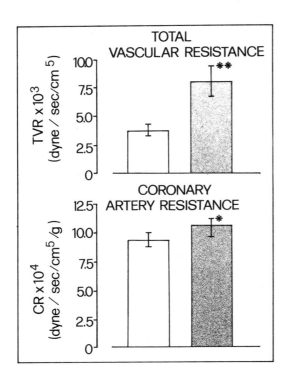

Fig. 10. Effect of methoxamine plus bleeding on total vascular resistance (TVR) and coronary resistance (CR). [* = difference from control group, p < 0.05; ** = difference from control group, p < 0.01].

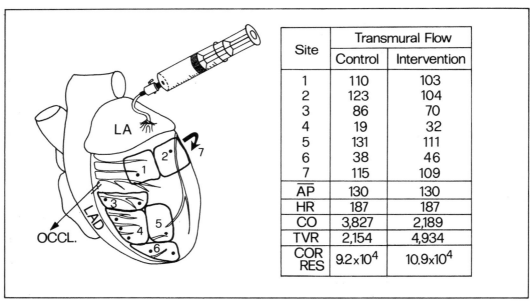

Site	Transmural Flow	
	Control	Intervention
1	110	103
2	123	104
3	86	70
4	19	32
5	131	111
6	38	46
7	115	109
$\overline{AP}$	130	130
HR	187	187
CO	3,827	2,189
TVR	2,154	4,934
COR RES	9.2×10^4	10.9×10^4

Fig. 11. An example illustrating the changes in regional myocardial blood flow measured by microsphere injection 15 min after coronary occlusion (control) and after 15 min of methoxamine + bleeding (intervention). [LA: left atrium; LAD: left anterior descending coronary artery; Occl: site of occlusion: $\overline{AP}$ mean arterial pressure; HR: heart rate; CO: cardiac output; TVR: total vascular resistance; Cor Res: coronary resistance]. Note the reduction of flow in the non-ischaemic areas (sites 1, 2, 3, 5 and 7) and its increase in the ischaemic areas (sites 4 and 6).

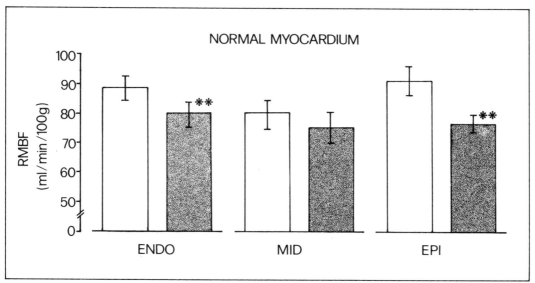

Fig. 12. Effects of coronary vasoconstriction by methoxamine on regional myocardial blood flow (RMBF) in normally perfused areas. [** = difference from control, p. < 0.01].

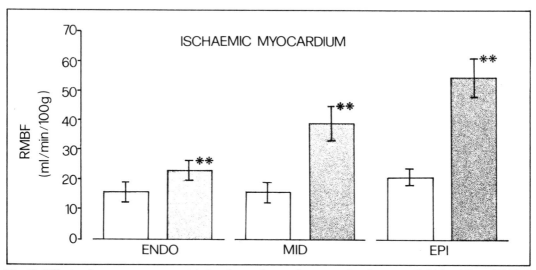

Fig. 13. Effects of coronary vasoconstriction by methoxamine on regional myocardial blood flow (RMBF) measured by the microspheres method in the ischaemic areas. Note the marked increase in collateral flow to these zones following the vascular constriction of the normal areas. [** = difference from control, p < 0.01].

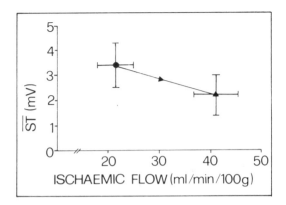

Fig. 14. Simultaneous changes in average ST segment elevation (ST) and ischaemic transmural flow, produced by the methoxamine-induced vasoconstriction. The coronary constriction produced an increase in collateral flow and consequently a reduction in ST.

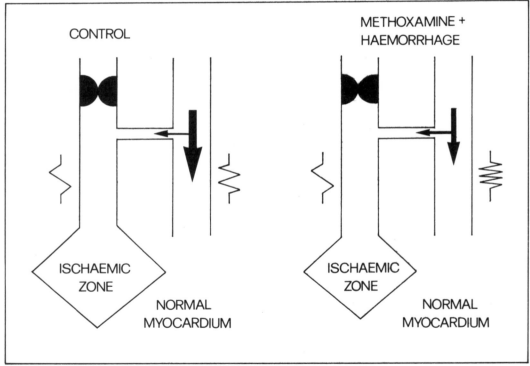

Fig. 15. Schematic representation of the hypothesis of reverse coronary steal. The left panel illustrates the distribution of flow following coronary artery occlusion. Blood flow in the non-occluded vessels is directed mainly to the normal myocardium (larger arrows), which exhibits a normal resistance; less blood flow (small arrows) is directed through the collaterals to the ischaemic areas (diamond shape), where the resistance is low (loose spring). The right panel illustrates the alterations due to methoxamine accompanied by bleeding. There is an increase in coronary resistance in the normal myocardium (tight spring), producing a decrease in flow to the normal myocardium (arrow of reduced size). Consequently, there is an increase in blood supply to the ischaemic zone (small arrow increases) through the collaterals and the extent of myocardial injury is reduced (smaller diamond).

References

1. Rona, G., Chappel, C.L. Balazs, T. and Gaudry, R.: An infarct-like myocardial lesion and other toxic manifestations produced by isoproterenol in the rat. *Arch. Path.*, 57, 443-455, 1959.
2. Wexler, B.C. and Kittinger, G.W.: Myocardial necrosis in the rat: serum enzymes, adrenal steroids and histopathological alterations. *Circ. Res.*, 13, 159-171, 1963.
3. Genovese, A., Chiariello, M., Ferro G., Cacciapuoti, A.A. Condorelli. M.: Myocardial hypertrophy in the rat. Correlation between two experimental models. *Jap. Heart J.*, 21, 511-528, 1980.
4. Waldeström. A., Hjalmarson, A., Thornell, L.: A possible role of noradrenaline in the development of myocardial infarction. Experimental study in isolated rat heart. *Am. Heart J.*, 95, 43, 1978.
5. Genovese, A., Chiariello, M., De Alfieri, W., Modesti, A. and Condorelli, M.: Myocardial enzymatic and morphologic changes by tyramine-released catecholamines in the rat. *J. Mol. Cell. Cardiol.*, Suppl. 1, 31, 1981.
6. Maroko, P.R. Kjekshus, J.K. Sobel, B.E., Wetanabe, T., Covell, J.W., Ross, J.Jr Braunwald, E.: Factors influencing infarct size following coronary artery occlusion. *Circulation*, 43, 67, 1971.
7. Libby, P., Maroko, P.R., Covell, J.W., Malloch, C.I., Ross J., Jr., Braunwald, E.: Effects of practolol on the extent of myocardial ischemic injury after experimental coronary occlusion and its effects on ventricular function in the normal and ischemic heart. *Cardiovas. Res.*, 7, 167. 1973.
8. Viloner, R.A., Fishbein, M.C., Braunwald, E., Maroko, P.R.: Effect of propranolol on mitochondrial morphology during acute myocardial ischemia. *Am. J. Cardiol.*, 41, 880, 1978.
9. Opie, L.H., Thomas, M.: Propranolol and experimental myocardial infarction. Substrate effects. *Postgrad. Med. J.*, 52, Suppl. 4, 124, 1976.
10. Mueller, H.S., Ayres, S.M., Religa, A. and Evans, R.G.: Propranolol in the treatment of acute myocardial infarction. Effects on myocardial oxygenation and hemodynamics. *Circulation*, 49, 1078, 1974.
11. Viloner, R.A., Fishbein, M.N., Cotran, R.S., Braunwald, E., Maroko, P.R.: The effect of propranolol on myocardiael injury in acute myocardial ischemia. *Circulation*, 55, 872, 1977.
12. Shell, W.E., Sobel, B.E.: Protection of jeopardized ischemic myocardium by reduction of ventricular afterload. *N. Engl. J. Med.*, 291, 482, 1974.
13. Skinner, C., Gaddie, J., Palmer, K.N.V.: Comparison of intravenous AH 5158 (ibidomide) and propranolol in asthma. *Br. Med. J.*, 2, 59, 1975.
14. Metha, J., Cohn, J.N.: Haemodynamic effect of labetalol, an alpha and beta-adrenergic blocking agent, in hypertensive subjects. *Circulation*, 55, 370, 1977.
15. Chiariello, M., Brevetti, G., De Rosa, G., Acunzo, R., Petillo, F., Rengo, F., Condorelli, M.: Protective effect of simultaneous alpha and beta-adrenoceptor blockade on myocardial cell necrosis after coronary arterial occlusion in rats. *Am. J. Cardiol.*, 46, 249, 1980.
16. Maclean, D., Fishbein, M.N., Braunwald, E., Maroko, P.R.: Long-term preservation of ischemic myocardium after experimental coronary artery occlusion. *J. Clin. Invest.*, 61, 541, 1978.
17. Fam, W.M., McGregor, M.: Effects of coronary vasodilator drugs on retrograde flow in areas of chronic myocardial ischemia. *Circ Res.*, 15, 355, 1974.
18. Rowe, G.G.: Inequalities of myocardial perfusion in coronary artery disease ("coronary steal"). *Circulation*, 42, 193, 1970.
19. Parratt, J.R., Ledingham, M.A., McArdloe, C.S.: Effect of a coronary vasodilator drug (carbochromen) on blood flow and oxygen extraction in acute myocardial infarction. *Cardiovasc. Res.*, 7, 401, 1973.
20. Shaper, W., Lewy., P., Flameng, W., Gijpen, L.: Myocardial steal produced by coronary vasodilation in chronic coronary artery occlusion. *Basic Res. Cardiol.*, 68, 3, 1972.
21. Chiariello, M., Gold, H.K. Leinbach, R.C., Davis, M.A., Maroko P.R.: Comparison between the effects of nitroprusside and nitroglycerin on ischemic injury during acute myocardial infarction. *Circulation*, 54, 766, 1976.
22. Gold, H.K., Chiariello, M., Leinbach, R.C., Davis, M.A., Maroko, P.R.: Deleterious effects of nitroprusside on myocardial injury during acute myocardial infarction. *Herz*, 1, 161, 1976.
23. Chiariello, M., Ribeiro, L.G.T., Davis, M.A. Maroko, P.R.: "Reverse coronary steal" induced by coronary vasoconstriction following coronary artery occlusion in dogs. *Circulation*, 56, 809, 1977.

Hypertension, recent advances and research
edited by M. Condorelli, A. Zanchetti
Cortina International, Verona 1982

The protective effect of Labetalol on the response to atrial pacing in coronary artery disease

G. BREVETTI, M. CHIARIELLO, G. VIGORITO, G. LAVECCHIA, S. VERRIENTI

Institute of Medical Pathology, University of Naples, Italy

Key words. Labetalol; Atrial Pacing; Coronary Artery Disease; Ischaemic Heart Diseases; Stress Tests; Beta-blockers; Myocardial Oxygen Consumption; Peripheral Resistances; Haemodynamic Measurements; Ventricular Afterload; Rate-Pressure Product; Left Ventricular End-Diastolic Pressure; Systemic Vascular Resistance; Left Ventricular Stroke Work Index; Selective Coronary Arteriography.

Summary. A haemodynamic study conducted during stress on 7 patients suffering from ischaemic heart diseases enabled us to demonstrate that, in contrast to what is commonly observed with the use of beta-blockers, the saving in oxygen consumption on the part of cardiac muscle is obtained without prejudice to myocardial performance.

In point of fact, the stroke volume and cardiac output values obtained at maximum stress after i.v. administration of Labetalol were substantially identical to those recorded during control exercise.

Similarly, no significant variations were observed in dp/dt/LVEDP, which constitutes a reliable index of myocardial oxygen consumption.

The significant decrease in peripheral resistances, and thus in afterload, observed after Labetalol, would definitely appear to be the decisive haemodynamic factor in the therapeutic action of the drug.

Introduction

Atrial pacing is well documented as a valid and reproducible stress test in patients with myocardial ischaemia and has been widely-used in these patients to assess the efficacy of therapeutic interventions [1-4].

Labetalol is the only drug having the characteristic of blocking both alpha- and beta-adrenergic receptors [5, 6]. In animal and human studies this drug has been found to decrease systemic vascular resistance and, thus, arterial pressure, with only a moderate slowing-down of heart rate [7-10]. According to this haemodynamic profile. Labetalol has been successfully employed in the treatment of hypertension [10-12]. However, the decrease in heart rate and myocardial contractility mediated by beta-block and the decline in ventricular afterload obtained by alpha-block, both resulting in a reduction in myocardial oxygen consumption, suggests that this drug could be beneficial also in coronary artery disease.

Accordingly, this study examines the haemodynamic effects of a single, intravenous dose of Labetalol in seven patients with myocardial ischaemia using atrial pacing as a stress.

Methods

Patients

Haemodynamic investigations with subsequent selective coronary arteriography and left ventriculography were performed in 7 male patients aged 43-58 years. All patients were in sinus rhythm and had stable exertional angina pectoris that could be reproduced during the bicycle ergometer stress test. One patient had sustained a previous myocardial infarction two years before the study. Three of the 7 were hypertensive, having systolic blood pressure above 150 mmHg, but only one had diastolic blood pressure exceeding 95 mmHg. The haemodynamic and angiographic details of each patient are reported in Table 1. None was receiving anti-hypertensive therapy or digoxin at the time of the study. All of the patients had been treated with long-acting nitrates, but they had not taken these drugs for at least 7 days before the investigation. Sublingual nitroglycerin was the only medication taken during the 7 days before the study, and it was discontinued on the morning of the study.

Written consent was obtained from each patient after the nature and the goals of the study had been fully explained.

Description of pacing technique

The pacing rate was started at 100 bmp (with the exception of patient 4, in whom the starting atrial pacing rate was 120 bpm) and increased by 10 bmp every 90 seconds until the onset of angina, the occurrence of noncapture or a rate of 150 bpm was achieved. When the patient experienced anginal pain during pacing, the pacing was continued at that rate for an average of 2-3 minutes to allow haemodynamic measurements. Thereafter, pacing was discontinued and pressures recorded in the immediate post-pacing period.

Study protocol

Patients were studied in a fasting state under premedication with diazepam, 5 mg p.o.. Under local anaesthesia, right heart catheterization was performed via a medial antecubital vein, while left heart catheterization, ventriculography and coronary arteriography were performed via a brachial artery. A 5 French bipolar catheter electrode was introduced through a second antecubital vein and positioned in the right atrium, in a stable pacing site.

The protocol of the study was the following: the patient rested for 15 minutes after instrumentation, and during the final 2-3 minutes of the conrol period (C_1) haemodynamic measurements were performed. Pacing (PC_1) was then started as described above and further records of pressures and cardiac output were obtained at the end-point. Pacing was then discontinued and pressures recorded in the immediate post-pacing period. After a 20-minute recovery period, rest haemodynamics were again measured (C_2) and thereafter Labetalol, 0.6 mg/kg, was administered i.v.. Five minutes later, new resting haemodynamics were assessed (L) and the pacing protocol was repeated as before (PC_2). At the end of the investigation, diagnostic selective coronary arteriography and left ventriculography were performed.

Haemodynamic measurements

Aortic and left ventricular end-diastolic pressure (LVEDP) were measured by a fluid-filled manometer using Statham P23Db pressure transducers and recorded on an OTE Biomedica preamplifier. Systolic and diastolic pressures were calculated by averaging individual systolic and diastolic points for at least 5 beats. Cardiac output was determined by the thermodilution technique using a Swan-Ganz

Table I. *Clinical and angiographic data.*

Patient	Age	Sex	Arterial pressure LVSP	(mmHg) MAP	Heart rate (b.p.m)	Previous myocardial infarction	Coronary LAD System	artery Circumflex system	obstruc-tion % RCA	Lv asynergy
1	58	M	107	75	60	—	75	50	50	+
2	47	M	120	83	81	—	—	75	—	+
3	50	M	117.5	90	71	—	75	—	50	—
4	43	M	205	142.5	98	+	75	—	—	+
5	52	M	200	105	60	—	75	50	—	—
6	58	F	150	102	73	—	—	50	50	—
7	52	M	120	116.6	66	—	75	50	50	+

110

Edwards catheter for thermodilution placed in the main pulmonary artery and an Edwards 9500 Cardiac Output Computer. The Lehman catheter placed in the aorta for pressure measurements was introduced into the left ventricle at various stages of the investigation to measure LVEDP and the first derivative of left ventricular pressure (dp/dt max); this latter index was recorded through a modular preamplifier for differential operations. Heart rate was derived from the electrocardiogram (Lead II) continuously monitored during the study. From the haemodynamic data, systemic vascular resistance was calculated according to the formula:

$$SVR = \frac{(MAP - right\,atrial\,pressure)}{Co} \times 80\ dynes/sec/cm^{-5}$$

where MAP indicates mean arterial pressure and CO, cardiac output. Left ventricular stroke work index (LVSWI) in g-m/m2 was calculated using the formula:

$$LVSWI = \frac{SI \times (MAP - LVEDP) \times 1.36}{100}$$

where SI stands for stroke index. The rate pressure product (RPP) was calculated as the product of systolic arterial pressure and heart rate.

Statistical analysis

All numbers in the paper are expressed as mean ± standard deviation. Statistical analysis was performed using Student's "t" test for paired samples.

Results

The clinical, haemodynamic and angiographic details of each patient are reported in Table 1. None of the patients included in the study presented any side effects as a consequence of i.v. administration of Labetalol.

Effects of atrial pacing before Labetalol

Three patients (Nos. 1, 3, and 7) experienced anginal pain during the atrial pacing performed before Labetalol administration. In patient 5 who did not develop angina, atrial pacing was stopped at 130 bpm on account of the development of 2:1 atrioventricular block. The rise in heart rate was associated with a significant fall in LVSWI from 54.1 ± 12.9 to 34.8 ± 10.6 g-m/m² ($p < 0.01$), and in stroke index from 49.8 ± 8.6 to 28.7 ± 5.9 ml/m² (p 0.01). Left ventricular systolic pressure and mean arterial pressure did not change during pacing, while LVEDP rose significantly from 14.6 ± 8.9 to 21.4 ± 10.3 mmHg ($p < 0.01$). The haemodynamic responses to pacing are shown in Table II.

Effects of Labetalol before pacing

The effects of Labetalol at rest are reported in Table III. The drug induced a significant decrease both in left ventricular systolic pressure ($p < 0.01$) and in mean arterial pressure ($p < 0.01$). Similarly, peripheral vascular resistance decreased from 1210 ± 221 to 1117 ± 200 dynes sec/cm/⁻⁵ ($p < 0.01$). Despite its beta-blocking action. Labetalol did not induce changes in heart rate, though dp/dt max fell from 1936 ± 400 to 1533 ± 413 ($p < 0.05$).

Table II. *Effects of atrial pacing before Labetalol.*

		LVSP (mmHg)	MAP (mmHg)	CI (ml/min/m²)	SI (ml/b/m²)	LVEDP (mmHg)	LVSWI (g-m/m²)	dp/dt (mmHg/sec)	SVR (dyn x sec x cm⁻⁵)
Control	mean	145.6	96.8	3673	49.8	14.6	54.1	1977	1163
	±SD	41.0	23.0	678	8.6	8.9	12.9	452	200
Pacing	mean	146.0	106.0	3701	28.7	21.1	34.8	1968	1267
	± S.D.	30.9	22.7	631	5.9	10.3	10.6	402	251
	P	n.s.	n.s.	n.s.	0.01	0.01	0.01	n.s.	n.s.

For meanings of abbreviations, see text.

Table III. *Response to intravenous Labetalol before atrial pacing.*

		LVSP (mmHg)	MAP (mmHg)	HR (b.p.m)	CI (ml/min /m²)	SI (ml/b/m²)	LVEDP (mmHg)	LVSWI (g-m/m²)	dp/dt (mmHg /sec)	SVR (dyn x sec x cm⁻⁵)
Before	mean	144.9	97.8	78.3	3571	46.7	14.9	51.0	1936	1210
Labetalol	±SD	29.7	16.3	18	459	10.6	10.1	9.1	436	221
After	mean	122.3	86.8	78.3	3248	42.8	14.2	41.4	1533	1117
Labetalol	±SD	21.3	15.8	18.6	451	10.5	7.0	11.2	413	200
	P	0.01	0.01	n.s.	n.s.	n.s.	n.s.	0.05	0.01	0.05

For meanings of abbreviations, see text.

Stroke index, cardiac index and LVEDP remained unmodified and a slight but significant decrease in LVSWI (p < 0.05) was observed.

Effects of Labetalol on the responses to atrial pacing

The effect of Labetalol on the responses to atrial pacing can be best appreciated when compared with those observed during similar stress prior to the administration.

a) Pain: whereas 3 patients developed ischaemic pain during pacing before Labetalol, none complained of chest pain following the drug administration. In patient 5, who developed 2:1 atrioventricular block during P_1, this conduction disturbance was observed at the same pacing rate as before during P_2, and, thus, pacing was discontinued.

b) Left ventricular systolic pressure and mean arterial pressure: after P_1, LVSP reached a value as high as 146.0 ± 30.9 mmHg, while after Labetalol, at the same pacing rate as before, it was 117.0 ± 23.6 mmHg, a value significantly (p < 0.01) lower than that recorded during P_1 (Fig. 11). Similarly, MAP was reduced by Labetalol from a control value of 106.0 ± 22.7 to 87.7 ± 21.1 mmHg (p < 0.05) (Fig. 1). The decrease in systolic pressure induced by Labetalol reflected a reduction in the double product (Fig. 1). Actually, it fell from a control value of 20267 ± 5092 to 16021 ± 3747 mmHg/min (p < 0.01).

c) Left ventricular performance: stroke index and cardiac index were not modified by Labetalol (Fig. 2). Stroke index was 28.7 ± 5.9 ml/beat/m² during P_1 and 26.8 ± 2.5 ml/be-

at/m² during P_2. Left ventricular end-diastolic pressure was slightly reduced by the drug from a control value of 21.4 ± 10.3 to 19.8 ± 8.1 mmHg during Labetalol pacing (Fig. 2). Similarly, dp/dt max remained unchanged (Fig. 2), while LVSWI decreased from 34.8 ± 10.6 to 26.9 ± 11.0 g-m/m² (p < 0.05).

d) Systemic vascular resistance: compared with P_1, there was a significant reduction in SVR during Labetalol pacing (Fig. 3). Actually, this parameter was reduced from a control value of 1267 ± 251 to 1028 ± 196 dynes/sec/cm⁻⁵ (p < 0.05).

Discussion

The results of this study demonstrate that the intravenous administration of Labetalol improved the pacing tolerance in patients with coronary artery disease mainly by decreasing left ventricular afterload. This is in agreement with previous studies demonstrating that Labetalol is able to enhance exercise capacity through a decrease in arterial pressure and double-product [9, 10, 13]. This haemodynamic effect may explain the disappearance of angina during Labetalol pacing in the 3 patients who experienced chest-pain during the first atrial pacing. The decreased afterload observed both at rest and during stress is probably related to the alpha-adrenergic blocking action of Labetalol [6, 8]. During pacing the peripheral vasodilator effect of this drug decreased mean aortic pressure, left ventricular stroke work index and double product, and thus the angina threshold.

112

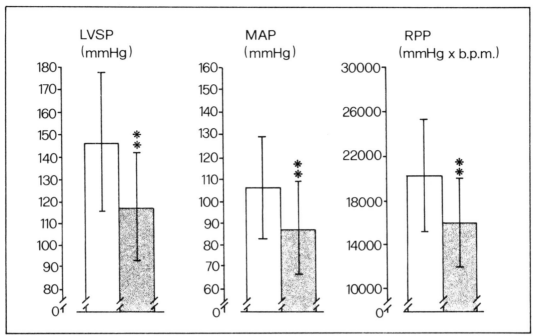

Fig. 1. Mean values (± SD) of left ventricular systolic pressure (LVSP), mean arterial pressure (MAP) and rate-pressure product (RPP) during atrial pacing before (solid columns) and after (striped columns) Labetalol. [** p < 0.01].

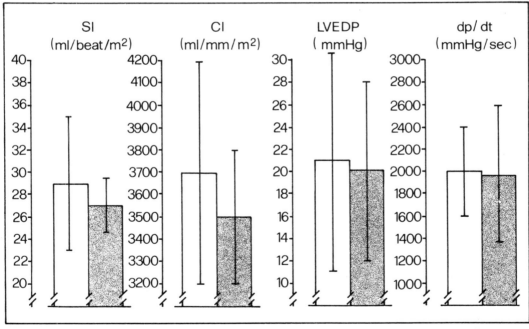

Fig. 2. Mean values (± SD) of stroke index (SI), cardiac index (CI), left ventricular end-diastolic pressure (LVEDP) and first derivative of left ventricular pressure (dp/dt) during atrial pacing before (solid columns) and after (striped columns) Labetalol.

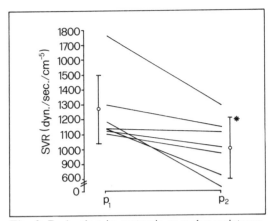

Fig. 3. Reduction in systemic vascular resistance induced by Labetalol during atrial pacing. [* p < 0.05. For meanings of abbreviations see text].

In addition to its alpha-blocking properties, Labetalol also exerts beta-blocking action; this is especially useful in limiting the reflex tachycardia which is elicited by peripheral vasodilation. Actually, in our study heart rate did not change at rest after Labetalol. Despite its beta-blocking properties, Labetalol did not increase LVEDP either at rest or during pacing. Left ventricular dp/dt max decreased at rest after Labetalol, but was unchanged during stress. These data suggest that Labetalol, unlike beta-blockers, is able to exert its protective effect on the ischaemic myocardium without significantly affecting left ventricular performance. The lack of effect of Labetalol on left ventricular function is probably related to is alpha-blocking property, which triggers off a reflex inotropic mechanism able to counterbalance the depressant effect exerted by beta-blockade on the myocardium. Therefore, Labetalol may have applicability in situations where other beta-adrenergic blocking drugs are contraindicated.

In a preliminary study carried out in normotensives with coronary heart disease, we demonstrated that the peak exercise heart rate, blood pressure and double product were significantly reduced with Labetalol, and these changes from placebo values were associated with an increase in exercise tolerance and a reduction in S-T segment depression [14]. Therefore, Labetalol appears an effective drug for patients with coronary artery disease; it is able to reduce myocardial oxygen demand with exercise, allowing the patient to perform more strenous external work.

Furthermore, since data on coronary blood flow were not available in this study, the possibility that improved oxidative metabolism secondary to either increased total flow or redistribution of flow to the ischaemic area cannot be clarified. Maxwell demonstrated that coronary blood flow was increased by intravenous administration of Labetalol in intact dogs; Chiariello et al. [15] demonstrated a markedly greater protective effect of Labetalol as compared to propranolol on myocardial cell necrosis after coronary artery occlusion in rats. These studies seem to support the hypothesis that Labetalol, with its alpha-adrenergic blocking properties, may increase coronary blood flow while also reducing myocardial oxygen demand. This issue, as well as the possibiliy that Labetalol on account of its alpha-blocking action may be useful in the prevention of coronary spasm, requires further investigation.

References

1. O'Brien K.P., Higgs L.M., Glancey D.L. Epstein S.E.: Haemodynamic accompaniments of angina. A comparison during angina induced by exercise and by atrial pacing. Circulation, 39, 735, 1969.
2. Balcon R., Hoy J., Malloy W., Sowton E.: Haemodynamic comparison of atrial pacing and exercise in patients with angina pectoris. Br. Heart J., 31, 168, 1969.
3. Chiong M.A., West R.O., Parker J.O.: Influence of nitroglycerin on myocardial metabolism and hemodynamics during angina induced by atrial pacing. Circulation, 45, 1044, 1972.
4. Chiong M.A., West R.O., Parker J.O.: The protective effect of glucose-insulin-potassium on the response to atrial pacing. Circulation, 54, 37, 1976.
5. Collier J.G., Dawnay N.A.H., Nachev C.H., Robinson B.P.: Clinical investigation of an antagonist at alpha and beta-adrenoceptors - AH 5158. Br. J. Pharmacol. 44, 286-93, 1972.
6. Farmer J.B., Kennedy I., Levy G.P., Marshall R.J.: Pharmacology of AH 5158: a drug which blocks both alpha and beta-adrenoceptors Br. J. Pharmacol., 45, 660-75, 1972.
7. Brittain R.T. and Levy G.P.: A review of the animal pharmacology of labetalol, a combined alpha and be-

ta-adrenoceptor blocking drug *Br. J. Clin. Pharmacol.*, 3, Suppl. 3, 681-94, 1976.

8. Richards D.A.: Pharmacological effects of labetalol in man *Br. J. Clin. Pharmacol.*, 3, Suppl. 3, 721-3, 1976.

9. Kock G.: Acute hemodynamic effects of an alpha and beta-receptor blocking agent (AH 5158) on the systemic pulmonary circulation at rest and during exercise in hypertensive patients. *Am. heart J.*, 93, 285-91, 1977.

10. Metha J. and Cohn J.N.: Hemodynamic effects of labetalol, an alpha and beta-adrenergic blocking agent in hypertensive subjects. *Circulation*, 55, 370-5, 1977.

11. Frick M.H., Pörsti P.: Combined alpha and beta-adrenoceptor blockade with labetalol in hypertension *Br. Med. J.*, 1, 1046-8, 1976.

12. Prichard B.N.C. and Boakes A.J.: Labetalol in long-term treatment of hypertension. *Br. J. Clin. Pharmacol.* 3, Suppl. 3, 743-50, 1976.

13. Richards D.A., Woodings E.P., Maconochie J.G.: Comparison of the effects of labetalol and propranolol in healthy men at rest and during exercise. *Br. J. Clin. Pharmacol.*, 4, 15-21, 1977.

14. Brevetti G., Chiariello M., Rengo F., Chiariello L., Paudice G., Lavecchia G., Condorelli M.: Labetalol in coronary artery disease. *VIII World Congress of Cardiology*, 17th-23rd September, 1978, Tokyo, Japan. Abstr. Book I, page 195. 1978.

15. Maxwell G.M.: Effects of alpha- and beta-adrenoceptor antagonist (AH 5158) upon general and coronary hemodynamics of intact dogs *Br. J. Clin. Pharmacol.*, 44, 370-2, 1973.

16. Chiariello M., Brevetti G., De Rosa G., Acunzo R., Petillo F., Rengo F., Condorelli M.: Protective effects of simultaneous alpha and beta-adrenergic receptor blockade on myocardial cell necrosis after coronary arterial occlusion in rats. *Circulation*, 46, 294-54, 1980.

Hypertension, recent advances and research
edited by M. Condorelli, A. Zanchetti
Cortina International, Verona 1982

Neural mechanisms in the pathophysiology of arterial hypertension

ALBERTO ZANCHETTI

Institute of Cardiovascular Research, University of Milan

Key words. Arterial Hypertension; Essential Hypertension; Experimental Hypertension; Hypertension-initiating Factors; Hypertension-maintaining Factors; Neural Mechanisms; Nervous Regulation of Circulation; Renal Mechanisms; Sympathetic Nervous System; Natriuresis; Resetting; Anti-hypertensive Drugs.

Summary. The distinction between neural mechanisms as hypertension-initiating and hypertension-maintaining factors, which proved so useful in experimental forms, is difficult to apply to the analysis of the clinical aspects of a disease such as essential hypertension, which may only very rarely be observed in the initial stage and which is generally studied in its advanced stages, when it is impossible or, at any rate, extremely hard to distinguish between primary and secondary factors.

The questions which we may pose in relation to arterial hypertension and, in particular, essential hypertension are the following: whether nervous regulation of the circulation is maintained in hypertension and, if so, what mechanisms make such preservation of regulation possible and to what extent nervous regulation is modified by the various anti-hypertensive drugs used in clinical practice.

The role of any mechanism which might be involved in such a complex disease of regulation as arterial hypertension has long been the subject of discussion and controversy. It is generally agreed that genetic factors are greatly important in determining blood pressure levels, but this statement, however important and correct, does not help to clarify the physiological mechanism through which inheritance influences blood pressure. It is also agreed that genetic factors must interact with environmental influences in order to significantly raise blood pressure, but there is no agreement on the identity or the importance of environmental factors. It would obviously be impossible to summarize all the aspects of the various controversies in a rather short review such as the present one. I shall limit myself to presenting and discussing some of the evidence concerning the involvement of the sympathetic nervous system and the possible relationship between nervous and renal factors in the development and maintenance of elevated blood pressure values.

Neural mechanisms

There is no doubt that the sympathetic nervous system represents a mechanism of primary importance in the regulation of circulation. The point is, however, whether sympathetic, or adrenergic, control is equally important in initiating or maintaining the derangement or those derangements of circulation that are defined as arterial hypertension.

Help in clarifying this confused matter may come, first of all, from a distinction between 1) an initiating role that nervous factors may play in certain types of experimental hypertension, as well as in some cases of human hypertension; and 2) a secondary role these mechanisms may play in coming on the scene later to maintain high blood pressure primarily raised by other factors.

In the field of experimental hypertension there is evidence both for types of hypertension initiated by neural mechanisms and for types of hypertension initiated by non-neural factors but maintained by sympathetic activity [1].

Experimental hypertension initiated neurally

One type of hypertension initiated neurally is represented by operant conditioning procedures which consist in conditioning an animal to perform in such a way as to avoid a painful stimulus or to obtain a reward. By prolonged daily sessions of operant conditioning for several weeks and months, Herd et al. [2] and Forsyth & Harris [3] have found that arterial pressure rises to high values and is maintained elevated for several months.

Another ingenious behavioural model to study psychosocial factors in the production of experimental hypertension has been devised by Henry et al. [4]. When mice are raised in colonies the behaviour of the various males rapidly differentiates: some, the dominant ones, develop a kind of aggressive behaviour, and prevent the other males from approaching the females and the nests. It has been shown that dominant male mice develop a sustained rise in blood pressure.

The same occurs for males raised in isolation, who are successively put into a large colony and fight prolongedly to establish their territory. All these mice develop hypertension, and - interestingly enough - they show a conspicuous increase in the catecholamine-synthesizing enzyme tyrosine hydroxylase in the adrenal medulla (which can be taken as a sign of increased adrenergic sympathetic activity). Even more interesting is the fact that socially stimulated hypertensive mice show an elevated incidence of aortic arteriosclerosis.

Strictly related to the behavioural work just summarized are the beautiful studies performed by Folkow and his group on spontaneous hypertensive rats of the Japanese strain [5].

Their experiments indicate that proneness to exaggerated defence reactions might play an important role in the development of the spontaneous hypertension of the rat. The pressor and heart rate increases in response to a stressful stimulus are much greater in spontaneously hypertensive rats than in normotensive comparisons, and this is true also for young SHRs during the early "pre-hypertensive" stage, but does not occur in renovascular hypertensive rats. These observations strongly suggest that in spontaneously hypertensive rats normal environmental stimuli interact with an inherent hyperreactivity of the defense mechanisms and that the more frequent and powerful neurogenic pressure rises contribute to the development of so-called "spontaneous" hypertension.

There is another strain of rats raised by Dahl that develop hypertension if exposed to a high-salt diet. It is interesting that in these rats an approach-avoidance conflict can take the place of salt intake as the immediate cause of hypertension [16]. All these experiments stress the important interaction between genetic and environmental factors in the development of hypertension.

Neural mechanisms in the maintenance of experimental hypertension

As I have mentioned earlier, there is also evidence that several types of experimental hypertension, clearly initiated by non-neural mechanisms, are nonetheless maintained by sympathetic activity.

We have shown that in the cat there is a stage of natural sleep, called desynchronized sleep, in which sympathetic activity is temporarily depressed, and this depression is particularly relevant when the animal has previously been subjected to interruption of the sino-aortic reflex [7]. Cats with renovascular hypertension and denervation of the sino-aortic reflex were studied during the wakefulness-sleep cycle [8]. Their blood pressure was markedly elevated during quiet wakefulness, but suppression of sympathetic activity during desynchronized sleep brought arterial pressure down to such low levels that the cat could no longer be defined as hypertensive.

Further evidence on the role of the sympathetic system in various types of experimental hypertension has been obtained by another approach. The drug, 6-hydroxydopamine, is actively taken up by noradrenergic nerve endings and makes them degenerate. Intracisternal injection of 6-hydroxydopamine destroys noradrenergic neurones in the brain stem responsible for vasoconstrictor tone. This procedure prevents the appearance of various types of experimental hypertension or markedly reduces the high blood pressure when hypertension has already developed [9].

When injected systemically, 6-hydroxydopamine provides a very effective means for inducing peripheral sympathectomy by destroying the noradrenergic endings of post-ganglionic sympathetic neurones. Chemical sympathectomy, combined or not with adrenalectomy, abolishes or prevents various types of experimental hypertension, even those initiated by non-neural factors such as DOCA and salt, or renovascular hypertensions [9].

Quite recently, Brody has shown that destruction of a region of the anterior hypothalamus (AV3V area) also prevents the development of renovascular and DOCA-salt hypertensions [10]. The AV3V region contains neurones of the lower brain stem that are destroyed by 6-hydroxydopamine.

How hypertension induced by primary interventions on non-neural mechanisms may result in central and peripheral activation of the sympathetic system is not clear. As far as DOCA and salt are concerned, data are available showing a relationship between sodium intake and noradrenaline storage and turnover [1]. Regarding renovascular hypertension, angiotensin II has been shown to exert various excitatory actions on the sympathetic system both centrally and peripherally [9].

Neural mechanisms in human hypertension

The useful distinction between initiating and maintaining factors we have made in discussing experimental hypertension is unfortunately more difficult to make with human essential hypertension, a condition that can hardly be studied at its beginning, and is most often observed in an already advanced stage when it is impossible or exceedingly conjectural to distinguish between primary and secondary factors.

What we can ask ourselves about neural mechanisms in human essential hypertension is whether nervous control of the circulation is maintained in the hypertensive subject, and by which mechanism or mechanisms sympathetic activity is preserved or altered in the presence of hypertension [12].

If we accept the physiological notion that vasoconstrictor sympathetic activity is under the powerful inhibitory control of sino-aortic baroreceptor reflexes, an increase in arterial pressure should lead, as a necessary consequence, to a depression and, if the elevation of pressure is marked, to the total suppression of sympathetic activity itself.

These considerations have directed the attention of the investigators to the possibility that baroreceptor reflexes are modified in hypertension.

Modifications of baroreceptor reflexes in experimental hypertension have been described under the term of resetting since the paper by McCubbin, Green and Page [12], who established that in the renovascular hypertensive dog the activity of the carotid sinus nerve fibres is smaller in spite of the fact that the existing arterial pressure is higher.

When studied in man, resetting can only be defined as resetting of the reflex response as a whole, and has been studied extensively by several authors, in particular by Sleight and his group and by Korner and his group [13, 14] as the heart rate response to brief changes in arterial pressure induced by drugs. As a result of these studies, Sleight and his colleagues have introduced the concept that baroreceptor sensitivity is decreased in human hypertension. The elegant technique employed by Sleight allows us to investigate arterial baroreceptor influences on heart rate and other cardiac functions, but obviously it cannot offer any direct information on the reflex control of peripheral circulation and blood pressure. In arterial hypertension, however, it is the study of baroreflex control of blood pressure that really matters, and we have recently developed a technique suitable for such a study, the variable pressure neck chamber. [15]

The variable pressure neck chamber consists of a collar made of plastic material encircling the neck from the shoulders to a plane approximately intersecting the lower part of the face and the skull, so that alterations in transmural pressure are evenly produced around the whole circumference of the neck arteries. Each end of the collar is provided with a double rubber valve system which allows the pneumatic pressure inside to be changed - not only in a positive direction; this makes it possible to produce a reduction as well as an increase in carotid transmural pressure; since carotid transmural pressure is the stimulus for activation of baroreceptors, these manoeuvres will result in a reduction and, respectively, in an increase in carotid sinus baroreceptor activity.

Figure 1 illustrates the differences in the baroreflex responses we observed in one group of normotensive subjects and in two groups of hypertensive patients, who were arbitrarily subdivided into "moderate" or "severe" hypertensives according to their basal arterial pressure [16-18].

In this graph the abscissae represent the changes in carotid transmural pressure which are induced by the neck chamber above and below the existing mean blood pressure; the ordinates represent the reflex responses, either increases or decreases in pressure. It is clear that major differences existed between the reflex functions in the normotensive subjects and in the two groups of hypertensive patients. The pressor response to reduction in carotid transmural pressure was maximal in the normotensive group, and decreased progressively in the group of moderate and in the group of severe hypertensives. However, the depressor response to increased carotid transmural pressure showed an almost exactly opposite pattern of change: it was minimal in normotensive subjects, and increased progressively to achieve its maximal value in the group with severe hypertension.

The lower part of Figure 1 describes the resetting of the baroreflex in hypertension by drawing stimulus-response curves for the carotid baroreceptors, that is by representing how much the baroreceptors increase their discharge when carotid pressure increases, and vice

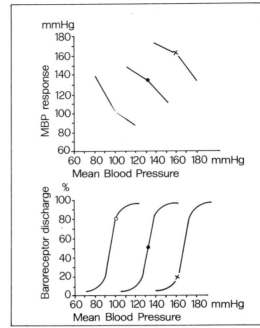

Fig. 1. *Top*, changes in mean arterial blood pressure (MBP) in response to changes in carotid sinus transmural pressure in normotensive subjects (open circle), those with moderate hypertension (closed circle) and those with severe hyperthension (cross). *Bottom*: curves represent the resetting of the carotid sinus baroreceptors in the three groups. [18]

versa. Our data can be interpreted by suggesting that in normotensives resting blood pressure is already capable of inducing a near-maximal activation of baroreceptor discharges; therefore, there will be little further increase in baroreceptor activity if pressure rises and the resulting reflex depressor response will be small; on the contrary, a fall in blood pressure will be able to decrease the already elevated baroreceptor discharge and to raise blood pressure considerably. In hypertensive patients the stimulus represented by resting blood pressure becomes progressively less and less effective in stimulating the baroreceptors and, in severe cases, it is just above the threshold for baroreceptor activation; consequently, a decrease in carotid sinus pressure can only slightly reduce the already low baroreceptor activity and the reflex increase in arterial pressure is small; but an increase in carotid pressure has wide possibilities for further increasing baroreceptor discharge and for reflexly reducing arterial pressure.

The physiopathologic meaning of baroreflex resetting in hypertension is that, despite the higher arterial pressure, there is less baroreceptor activity to inhibit sympathetic tone, and arterial pressure can therefore be maintained by sympathetic vasoconstrictor tone, and the elevated level of sympathetic activity can be easily inhibited when baroreceptors are stimulated.

This is the reason why the hypertensive patient can modulate his sympathetic activity during everyday life, and show adequate cardiovascular responses during exercise, stress, etc. This is the reason why so many drugs acting on the sympathetic nervous system are capable of lowering arterial pressure in the majority of hypertensive patients [11].

Recent technical developments have provided better means by which we can measure the considerable changes in arterial pressure occurring mostly through neural mechanisms, during both day and night in hypertensive patients. These recent developments consist in methods for continuously and directly recording blood pressure for extended (24- or 48-hour) periods while the patient is performing undisturbed.

The technique we are using [19] was initially developed by Littler and Sleight in Oxford [20]. A thin catheter (10 to 15 cm long, 1.2 mm inner diameter) is introduced into a radial artery under sterile precautions following local anaesthesia. The catheter is connected, through a tubing fixed to the forearm, to a miniaturized pressure transducer within a plastic box fixed to the chest at the level of the right atrium. The output of the transducer is fed into the direct-current amplifier of a miniaturized battery-supplied tape recorder fixed around the waist. Integral parts of the apparatus are a 40 ml saline reservoir and a small constant-flow pump which keeps the catheter open by continuous washing at a very low rate. The tape cassette allows continuous recording of the arterial pressure signal for 24 hrs without interference from the physician.

An example of a 24-hr blood pressure recording in a patient with essential hypertension of moderate severity is shown in Figure 2. There are considerable fluctuations in arterial pressure, with rises and falls, and the behavioural correlates of these blood pressure modifications can often be identified by observation of the patient or by signalling with a marker on the tape record various events during his daily life.

The prolonged fall in pressure occurring during night hours is known to be due to sleep. Another fall can be seen between hours 14 and 16, due to the healthy Italian habit of taking a siesta. It is interesting to see how the decrease in sympathetic tone during sleep reduces blood pressure in human hypertension, just as we have shown happens in the hypertensive animal.

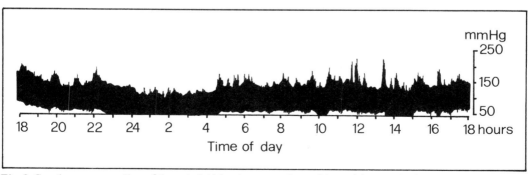

Fig. 2. Continuous recording of the arterial blood pressure in a subject with essential hypertension, using the Oxford technique. The recording began at 6 p.m. and terminated at 6 p.m. the following day.[19]

121

Renal mechanisms

The hypothesis that the kidney, through the derangement of one or another of its functions, plays a fundamental rôle in initiating and maintaining hypertension has long been a favorite one among investigators of hypertension since the first description of hypertension in glomerulonephritis by Bright in 1836, through the work of Volhard in the first quarter of this century down to the recent conception so forcibly emphasized by Guyton.

According to Guyton's conception [21], in the normal kidney the relation between arterial pressure and renal excretion of sodium is such that even a small increase in arterial pressure causes a very great increase in sodium excretion and this promptly and entirely corrects the rise in pressure. This phenomenon is called pressure natriuresis. This is the reason why Guyton defines the kidney as a pressure regulating mechanism with infinite gain. According to Guyton any non-renal factor, neural factors included, though capable of increasing blood pressure, can do this only transiently as pressure natriuresis would promptly nullify the initial rise in pressure. On the other hand, an alteration of the function of the kidney would cause sodium retention and lead to a permanent increase in pressure through a chain of events, summarized by Guyton as follows: increase in plasma volume, increase in cardiac output, and later development of increased vascular resistance through a phenomenon defined by Guyton as whole body autoregulation; the increased vascular resistance would then return toward normal along with both cardiac output and plasma volume.

There are very important aspects in Guyton's arguments but also some limitations.

The first important limitation consists in the fact that the hypothesis requires that, at least in a given stage, plasma volume and extracellular fluid volume are increased; while both these volumes are regularly found increased in primary aldosteronism and in hypertension due to renal failure, they are generally found to be slightly decreased, rather than increased, in essential hypertension.

Even if pressure natriuresis is a control mechanism with infinite gain, as stressed by Guyton, we should expect, at most, a return of volume to baseline values, not a reduction below baseline.

The second difficulty resides in the mechanisms responsible for an augmented cardiac output. It is certainly true that several authors have reported cardiac output to be somewhat elevated in some types of borderline hypertension, especially in the young, and that these light hypertensions might hypothetically represent an initial stage of essential hypertension. However, investigations performed by Julius [22] have shown that in subjects with borderline hypertension cardiac output becomes equal to that measured in normotensives after total blockade of cardiac innervation by propranolol and atropine. Therefore, the increase in cardiac output seems to result from autonomic disregulation rather than from an expansion of body volumes as required by Guyton's hypothesis.

A third difficulty results from observations by Lund-Johansen [23]. Basic to Guyton's concept of autoregulation is the hypothesis that autoregulation causes constriction of a vascular bed when flow to that organ is above its metabolic needs. Lund-Johansen has recently observed that young subjects with mild hypertension characterized by an augmented cardiac output also have a proportional increase in oxygen consumption, so that no disproportion can be found between whole body blood flow and metabolic requirements.

All these objections, or unsolved problems, do not mean, in my opinion, that pressure natriuresis is not an important phenomenon in hypertension. Figure 3 indicates that the role of the arterial pressure-sodium excretion curve in hypertension can be interpreted in two different ways [24]. On the left, the curve is shifted to the right and/or its slope depressed by a primary disturbance of renal sodium excretion or by some agent acting only on renal sodium excretion; as a consequence, there will be a transient phase of sodium retention and volume expansion, lasting until the consequent blood pressure increase will bring sodium excretion back to equilibrium: this is the mecha-

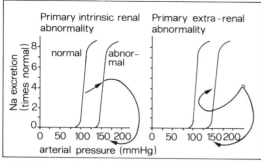

Fig. 3. Resetting of pressure-natriuresis curve A) by a primary renal mechanism; B) by a primary pressor system.

nism that can easily explain hypertension in renal insufficiency and in primary aldosteronism.

On the right, a primary pressor agent may both increase arterial pressure by means of diffuse vasoconstriction and simultaneously shift to the right and/or depress the renal excretion curve, thus preventing the primary blood pressure increase from being corrected by a large pressure natriuresis. This interpretation does not imply any phase - even a transient one - in which hypertension is accompanied by volume increase; the readjustment of renal function is only instrumental in preventing too great a reduction in plasma and extracellular fluid volume. This is what seems to occur in pheochromocytoma with continuous hypertension, in which volume contraction is a well-known characteristic; it may also be what occurs in essential hypertension, in which volumes are also decreased, though to a much smaller extent.

The sympathetic system is certainly possessed of several mechanisms by which renal function can be modified. One is renal vasoconstriction, particularly vasoconstriction of the afferent arteriole. The other mechanism is release of renin from juxtaglomerular cells. There is also mounting evidence that the renal nerves can influence water and sodium excretion from the kidney independently of vasomotor phenomena through a direct action on proximal tubular reabsorption (see [25]).

Figure 4 summarizes a hypothetical sequen-

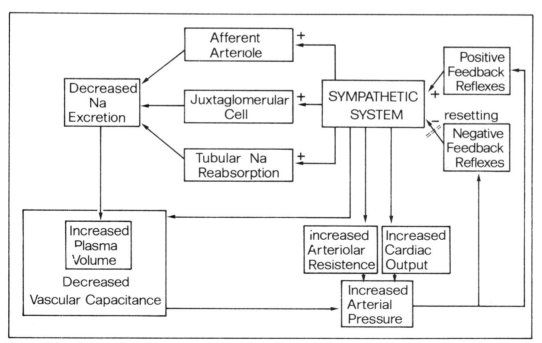

Fig. 4. Role of sympathetic system, cardiovascular reflexes, and sympathetic control of renal function in hypertension.[18]

ce of physiological events, leading to raised blood pressure. It is conceivable that sympathetic activity may be primarily increased either centrally or reflexly, through a primary resetting of negative feedback reflexes such as sinoaortic baroreflexes. Sympathetic activity by augmenting cardiac output and arteriolar resistance can reproduce the hemodynamic pattern characterizing essential hypertension, either borderline or established hypertension. Maintenance of sympathetic activity in spite of the increased blood pressure will be assured by further resetting of depressor reflexes, while pressure natriuresis will be reduced through the various mechanisms of sympathetic control of renal function. Eventually, as vascular hypertrophy develops, the participation of sympathetic activity in sustaining the hypertension might become less necessary.

This is, of course, just one of the many possible sequences of events that could lead to elevated blood pressure, and involving central and reflex sympathetic activity, the kidney, the heart and the vascular smooth muscle. Genetic factors play an important role in determining arterial pressure levels, but we still must learn at which level these factors intervene; if inheritance of blood pressure is polygenic, several functions may well be involved simultaneously or differently in different individuals. It remains to be more firmly established whether sympathetic activity and its reflex influences on the cardiovascular system are inherited and to what degree.

References

1. Zanchetti, A., Bartorelli, C.: Central nervous mechanisms in arterial hypertension: experimental and clinical evidence. In: J. Genest, E. Koiw, O. Kuchel, eds., *Hypertension*, New York, McGraw-Hill, 1977, p. 59.
2. Herd, J.A., Morse W.H., Kelleher, R.T., Jones, L.G.: Arterial hypertension in the squirrel monkey during behavioral experiments. *Am. J. Physiol.* 217, 24, 1969.
3. Forsyth, R.P., Harris, R.E.: Circulatory changes during stressful stimuli in Rhesus monkeys. *Circ. Res.* 26-27, Suppl. 1, 13, 1970.
4. Henry J.P., Stephens, P.M., Santisteban G.A.: A model of psychosocial hypertension showing reversibility and progression of cardiovascular complications. *Circ. Res.* 36, 156, 1975.
5. Folkow, B.: Central neurohormonal mechanisms in spontaneously hypertensive rats compared with human essential hypertension. *Clin. Sci. Mol. Med.* 48, Suppl. 2, 205, 1975.
6. Friedman, R., Iwai, J.: Genetic predisposition and stress-induced hypertension. *Science* 193, 161, 1976.
7. Mancia, G., Baccelli, G., Adams, D.B., Zanchetti, A.: Vasomotor regulation during sleep in the cat. *Am. J. Physiol.* 220, 1086, 1971.
8. Zanchetti, A., Baccelli, G., Guazzi, M., Mancia, G.: The effect of sleep in experimental hypertension. In: G. Onesti, K.E. Kim, J.H. Moyer, eds. *Hypertension: Mechanisms and Management* New York, Grune & Stratton, 1973, p. 133.
9. De Champlain, J.: Experimental aspects of the relationships between the autonomic nervous system and catecholamines in hypertension. In: J. Genest, E. Koiw, O. Kuchel, eds., *Hypertension*, New York, McGraw-Hill, 1977, p. 76.
10. Brody, M.J., Fink, G.D., Buggy, J., Haywood, J.R., Gordon, F.J., Johnson, A.K.: The role of the anteroventral third ventricle (AV3V) region in experimental hypertension. *Circ. Res.* 43, Suppl. 1, 1, 1978.
11. Zanchetti, A., Mancia, G.: Aspectos clínicos del control neurogénico de la circulacion en la hipertensiòn arterial. *Medicina, Buenos Aires*, 39, 71, 1979.
12. McCubbin, J.W., Green, J.H., Page, I.H.: Baroreceptor function in chronic renal hypertension. *Circ. Res.* 4, 205, 1956.
13. Sleight, P.: Reflex control of the heart rate. *Am. J. Cardiol.* 44, 889, 1979.
14. Korner, P.I., West M.J., Uther, J.B.: "Steady-state" properties of the baroreceptor-heart rate reflex in essential hypertension in man. *Clin. Exp. Pharmacol. Physiol.* 1, 65, 1974.
15. Ludbrook, J., Mancia, G., Ferrari, A., Zanchetti, A.: The variable-pressure neck chamber method for studying the carotid baroreflex in man. *Clin. Sci. Mol. Med.* 53, 165, 1977.
16. Mancia, G., Ferrari, A., Gregorini, L., Valentini, R., Ludbrook, J., Zanchetti, A.: Circulatory reflexes from carotid and extracarotid baroreceptor areas in man. *Circ. Res.* 41, 309, 1977.
17. Mancia, G., Ludbrook, J., Ferrari, A., Gregorini, L., Zanchetti, A.: Baroreceptor reflexes in human hypertension. *Circ. Res.* 43, 170, 1978.
18. Zanchetti, A.: Overview of cardiovascular reflexes in hypertension. *Am. J. Cardiol.* 44, 912, 1979.
19. Mancia, G., Zanchetti, A.: Continuous arterial blood pressure recording in human hypertension: A methodological approach. In: Hegyeli, R., ed. *Atherosclerosis Reviews*, Vol. 7: *Measurement and Control of Cardiovascular Risk Factors* New York, Raven Press, 1980, p. 247.
20. Littler, W.A., Honour, A.J., Sleight, P., Stott, F.D.: Continuous recording of direct arterial pressure and electrocardiogram in unrestricted man. *Br. Med. J.* 3, 76, 1977.
21. Guyton, A.C., Coleman, T.G., Cowley, A.W., Manning, R.D., Norman, R.A., Ferguson, J.D.: A systems analysis approach to understanding long-range arte-

rial blood pressure control and hypertension. *Circ. Res.* 35, 159, 1974.

22. Julius, S., Esler, M.D., Randall, O.S.: Role of the autonomic nervous system in mild human hypertension. *Clin. Sci. Mol. Med.* 40, Suppl. 2, 243, 1975.

23. Lund-Johansen, P. Haemodynamic effects of antihypertensive agents. In: E.D. Freis, ed., *The Treatment of Hypertension*, Lancaster, MTP Press Limited, 1978, p. 61.

24. Zanchetti, A., Mancia, G.: Baroreflexes in hypertension. In: *The Fundamental Fault in Hypertension. Proceedings of a Workshop Conference.* In press.

25. Zanchetti, A., Stella, A., Baccelli, G., Mancia, G.: Neural influences on kidney funtion in the pathogenesis of arterial hypertension. In: G. Onesti, C.R. Klimt, eds., Hypertension - *Determinants, Complications, and Intervention*, New York, Grune & Stratton, 1979, p. 99.

Hypertension, recent advances and research
edited by M. Condorelli, A. Zanchetti
Cortina International, Verona 1982

The cardioprotective and vascularprotective properties of Labetalol

D.A. RICHARDS

Glaxo Group Research Ltd., Ware, Hertfordshire

Key words. Labetalol; Cardioprotective Properties; Vascularprotective Properties; Clinical Pharmacology; Log-Dose Response Curves; Beta-adrenoceptor Blocking Effects; Alpha-adrenoceptor Blocking Effects; Alpha-beta-adrenoceptor Blocking Effects; Propranolol; Cold Stimulus; Cardiovascular Effects; Isoprenaline; Phenylephrine; Noradrenalin.

Summary. The clinical pharmacology of Labetalol has been evaluated using pharmacological and physiological test methods.

Labetalol displaces the log dose-response curves to the right of isoprenaline-induced increases in heart rate, cardiac output and decreases in diastolic BP. The similarity in the displacements of these curves suggests Labetalol has non-selective β-adrenoceptor-blocking properties.

Labetalol inhibitis exercise-induced increases in heart rate and systolic BP, inhibits tilt tachycardia and that associated with Valsalva's manoeuvre.

Labetalol displaces the log dose-response curves of phenylephrine and noradrenaline-induced increases in systolic and diastolic BPs to the right consistent with an α-adrenoceptor-blocking action.

Labetalol inhibits increases in BP due to a cold stimulus, whereas propranolol does not.

The combined α- and β-adrenoceptor-blocking effect of Labetalol after acute chronic administration leads to reductions in BP and peripheral resistance but little change in heart rate or cardiac output at rest. During exercise, increases in BP and heart rate are attenuated but cardiac output increases are only significantly diminished at high levels of exercise.

This paper reviews the pharmacological and haemodynamic effects of Labetalol in man and identifies possible benefits to hypertensive patients which may result from the use of Labetalol.

The pharmacological properties of Labetalol as identified in animal preparations were first described by Farmer et al. [1] in 1972. It was shown that this drug possessed both alpha- and beta-adrenoceptor blocking properties. Subsequently it has been shown that these same properties are also measurable in man[2, 5].

Beta-adrenoceptor blocking effects

Intravenously infused isoprenaline in man increases the heart rate and reduces the diastolic blood pressure in a dose-related manner due to beta$_1$- and beta$_2$-adrenoceptor stimulation. Labetalol antagonised these effects of isoprenaline and linear log-dose response curves of isoprenaline-induced increases in heart rate and reductions in diastolic blood pressure are shifted to the right after both oral and intravenous administration of Labetalol. The magnitude of the shift is similar for changes in heart rate and diastolic pressure and hence the beta-antagonistic effect of Labetalol is non-selective (Figs. 1 and 2) [2, 3].

Beta-adrenoceptor blocking drugs inhibit the increase in heart rate and systolic blood pressure induced by vigorous exercise. Labetalol administered orally or intravenously has a

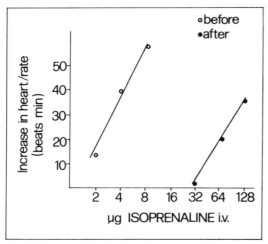

Fig. 1. Isoprenaline-induced increases in heart rate before and after intravenous Labetalol.

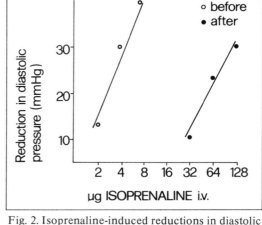

Fig. 2. Isoprenaline-induced reductions in diastolic pressure before and after intravenous Labetalol.

dose-related inhibitory effect upon exercise tachycardia and increases in systolic pressure [3-4] (Fig. 3). In comparison with propranolol where isoprenaline and exercise are used as the test methods, Labetalol has similar qualitative beta-antagonist properties but quantitatively differs from propranolol by a range of 4-6 fold in potency [6]. By contrast, however, where Labetalol and propranolol have been compared in respect of their effects upon airways func-

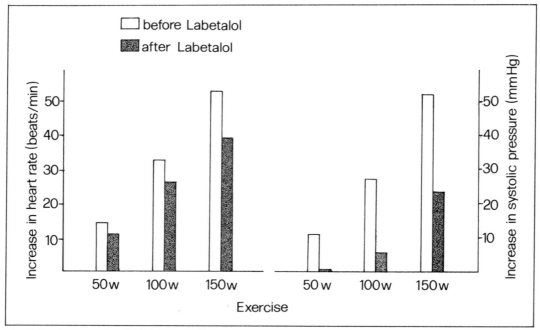

Fig. 3. During exercise, the inhibitory effects upon heart rate and systolic blood pressure in the same six subjects after Labetalol and propranolol were qualitatively similar.[6] However, unlike the effects observed after drugs such as propranolol, intravenous Labetalol (1.5 mg/kg) produced small reductions in diastolic pressure during exercise.[7] (Figure 20).

tion, the two drugs differ significantly from each other. Propranolol administered to normal healthy males significantly reduces peak expiratory flow both at rest and during exercise [6].

After Labetalol, however, no significant reduction occurred. In another study, propranolol reduced resting FEV_1 and that fall induced by inhaled histamine was enhanced whereas no such effects occurred with Labetalol [7]. Thus, there is a difference between Labetalol and propranolol in their effects upon the respiratory traet which have also been demonstrated in asthmatic patients [8].

Alpha-adrenoceptor blocking effects

Intravenously infused noradrenaline or phenylephrine increase systemic blood pressure in a dose-related manner due to alpha-adrenoceptor stimulation. Labetalol antagonises this effect and linear log-dose response curves of phenylephrine- phenylephrine and noradrenaline-induced increases in systolic blood pressure are shifted to the right after Labetalol administration (Fig. 4) [2, 5]. Noradrenaline infused intravenously has both alpha- and beta-stimulant effects though the predominant measurable effect is that mediated through alpha-adrenoceptors. It has been shown that Labetalol competitively antagonises the systolic and

diastolic pressure effects induced by noradrenaline but leaves unaffected the reflexly induced reduction of heart rate and cardiac output (Fig. 5) [9]. The alpha-adrenoceptor antagonist phentolamine has similar effects to that of Labetalol in this regard since it also antagonises noradrenaline-induced pressor responses [10]. Exposure to cold induced a pressor effect and it has been shown that immersing a hand in ice-cold water for 60 seconds elevates blood pressure in normotensive man. This effect seems to be mediated through alpha-adrenoceptors. Administration of propranolol did not prevent cold-induced increases in blood pressure but Labetalol had a significant inhibitory effect (Fig. 6) [7].

Cardiovascular effects of Labetalol

Administration of either oral or intravenous Labetalol in normotensive and hypertensive subjects results in an immediate reduction in systolic and diastolic blood pressure without significant reduction in heart rate or cardiac output. Labetalol reduces total peripheral resistance and its overall haemodynamic effect results from its combined alpha- and beta-blocking properties (Fig. 7) [9, 11]. In contrast, although alpha-blockade produced by phentolamine reduces blood pressure, heart rate and cardiac output are elevated due to reflex responses (Fig. 8). However, Labetalol's effect upon blood pressure is unaccompanied by cardiac stimulation.

Furthermore, acute beta blockade with propranolol does not cause a reduction in blood pressure but lowers both heart rate and cardiac output. Thus in respect of Labetalol it has been shown that the pattern of haemodynamic change induced by Labetalol is different from either an alpha- or a beta-blocker alone but the overall effect is similar to that of the combination of a vasodilator (hydralazine) plus a beta-blocker (propranolol) [11].

Discussion

Using well established test methods for identifying both alpha- and beta adrenoceptor blocking effects it has been shown that Labetalol possesses these properties in combina-

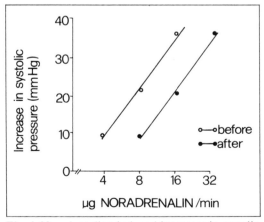

Fig. 4. Noradrenaline-induced increases in systolic blood pressure before and after intravenous Labetalol.

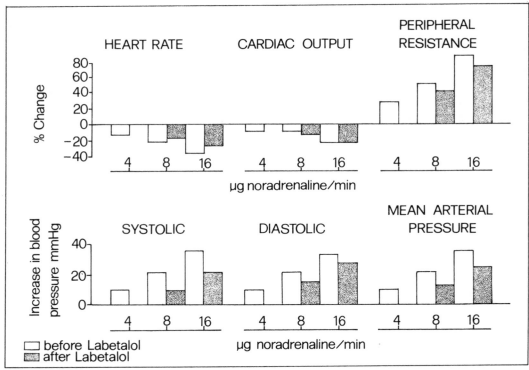

Fig. 5. Effects of Labetalol on noradrenaline-induced changes in haemodynamic indices.

tion. The resultant effect of blocking simultaneously alpha- and beta-adrenoceptors within the cardiovascular system in man is to produce a fall in blood pressure due to a reduction in total peripheral resistance but without producing significant reductions in heart rate or cardiac output. This overall effect differs therefore from the individual haemodynamic effects produced by alpha- or beta-blockade alone. It is well recognised that inducing a reduction in blood pressure by beta-blocking drugs administered chronically has also a "cardioprotective" effect in so far as exercise- or emotion-induced elevations in blood pressure and heart rate are significantly inhibited. In the case of Labetalol it is clear that its beta-adrenoceptor blocking effect prevents the usual cardiac stimulation which results from endogenous and exogenous stimuli. Thus Labetalol has "cardioprotective" properties.

In addition, however, the vasculature is probably protected further from hypertensive events in the case of Labetalol since it blocks those alpha-adrenoceptors through which sympathetically mediated vasoconstriction occurs. This is exemplified by the data which show that Labetalol inhibits cold-induced increases in blood pressure whereas propranolol, not possessing alpha-blocking activity, does not. Furthermore, it has been found in clinical use of Labetalol that patients who formerly suffered from symptoms of cold hands and feet on simple beta-blocking drugs either lose the symptoms entirely or find that they are modified.

Thus it seems that Labetalol may have a "vasculo-protective" effect. Since therefore Labetalol possesses cardioprotective and vasculoprotective properties resulting directly from its pharmacological effects, it would seem to be a

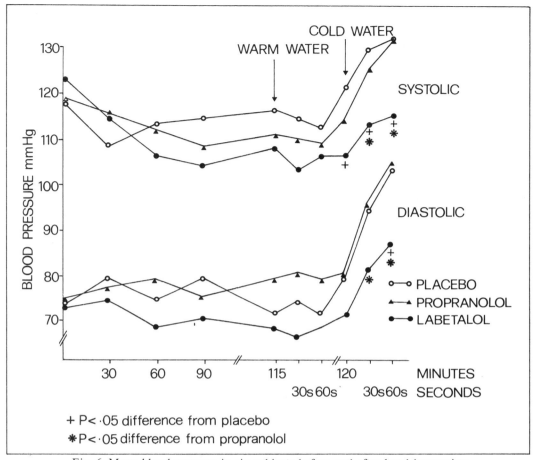

Fig. 6. Mean blood pressure in six subjects before and after hand immersion.

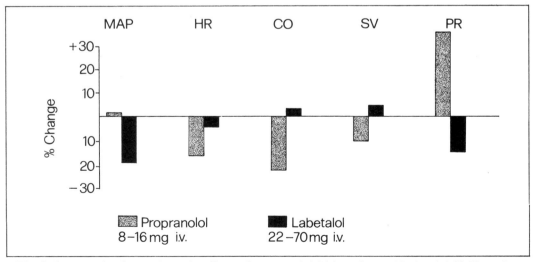

Fig. 7. Comparative haemodynamic effects of propranolol 8-16 mg i.v. and Labetalol 22-70 mg i.v.

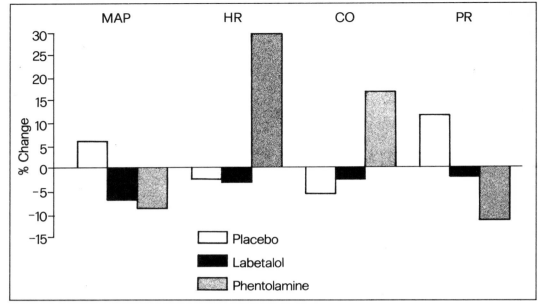

Fig. 8. Immediate haemodynamic effects of placebo, Labetalol and phentolamine.

most suitable choice for the treatment of hypertensive patients.

References

1. Farmer J.B., Kennedy I., Levy G.P., Marshall R.J.: Pharmacology of AH 5158, a drug which blocks both beta- and alpha-adrenoceptors. *Br. J. Pharmacol.* 45, 660-675, 1972.
2. Richards D.A.: Pharmacological effects of labetalol in man. *Br. J. Clin Pharmacol.* 3, Suppl. 721-723, 1976.
3. Richards D.A., Prichard B.N.C., Boakes A.J., Tuckman J., Knight E.J. Pharmacological basis for antihypertensive effects of intravenous labetalol. *Br. Heart J.* 39 99-106, 1977.
4. Richards D.A., Woodings E.P., Stephens M.D.B., Maconochie J.G.: The effects of oral AH 5158, a combined alpha- and beta-adrenoceptor antagonist in healthy volunteers. *Br.J. Clin. Pharmacol.* 1 506-510, 1974.
5. Richards D.A., Prichard B.N.C., Hernandez R.: Circulatory effects of noradrenaline and adrenaline before and after labetalol. *Br. J. Clin. Pharmacol.* 7 371-378, 1979.
6. Richards D.A., Woodings E.P., Maconochie J.G.: Comparison of the effects of labetalol and propranolol in healthy men at rest and during exercise. *Br. J. Clin. Pharmacol.* 4 15-21, 1977.
7. Maconochie J.G., Woodings E.P., Richards D.A.: Effects of labetalol and propranolol in histamine-induced bronchoconstriction in normal subjects. *Br. J. Clin. Pharmacol.* 4 157-162, 1977.
8. Skinner C., Gaddie J., Palmer K.N.V.: Comparison of intravenous AH 5158 (labetalol) and propranolol in asthma. *Br. Med. J.* 2 59-61, 1975.
9. Richards D.A., Prichard B.N.C., Dobbs R. J.: Adrenoceptor blockade of the circulatory responses to intravenous isoproterenol. *Clin. Pharmacol. Therap.* 24, 264-273, 1978.
10. Richards D.A., Woodings E.P., Prichard B.N.C.: Circulatory and alpha-adrenoceptor blocking effects of phentolamine. *Br. J. Clin. Pharmacol.* 5 507-513, 1978.
11. Prichard B.N.C., Thompson F.D., Boakes A.J., Jockes A.M.: Some haemodynamic effects of compound AH 5158 compared with propranolol, propranolol plus hydralazine and diazoxide: the use of AH 5158 in the treatment of hypertension. *Clin. Sci. Mol. Med.* 48, 97s-101s, 1975.

Treatment of hypertension with Labetalol: a multi-centre study

G. BREVETTI, M. CHIARIELLO, S. VERRIENTI, G. LAVECCHIA, F. RENGO

Institute of Medical Pathology, 2nd Medical School, University of Naples, Italy

with theco-operation of

Angrisani P. (Salerno), Brancaccio A. (Torre del Greco), Galloro V., Mayer M. (Napoli), Lanni N., Luongo M., Grimaldi U., Scaglione B. (Benevento), Lombardi S., Miele A. (Benevento), Carile L. (Larino), Giovine F. (Eboli), Mecca D., Caiazza F. (Potenza), Bray (Maglie), Brindicci G. (Bari), Coluccia L. (S. Cesareo), Nuzzolese V. (Altamura), Quinto V. (Corato), D'Amico N. (Catanzaro), Filocamo G. (Locri), Schirippa V., Attisano N. (Locri), Striano U. (Rossano Calabro), Vigna L. (Castrovillari), Bonaventura S., Lorenti J. (Lentini), Casella G., Pavia L. (Messina), Di Benedetto A. (Palermo), Ferraguto P., Salici G. (Augusta), Ferrari G., Nicoletti B. (Enna), Nastri L. (Agrigento), Pittera A. (Paternò), Rizza O. (Ragusa), Scapellato L., Stornello M. (Siracusa)

Key words. Labetalol; Mild Hypertension; Moderate Hypertension; Severe Hypertension; Multi-centre Trial; Side Effects; Computer Analysis; Diuretic.

Summary. A multi-centre Labetalol trial was carried out in 377 hypertensive patients in 28 hospital centres. The average duration of the study was 12 weeks. Computer analysis of the records of 277 patients who completed the study period showed that treatment resulted in good blood pressure control in 62.8% of cases and was particularly effective in those patients with mild-to-moderate hypertension. Supine systolic blood pressure was reduced by Labetalol from a control value of 186 ± 20 to 157 ± 21 mmHg ($p < 0.01$), diastolic from 107 ± 10 to 91 ± 12 mmHg ($p < 0.01$) and heart rate from 83 ± 10 to 74 ± 9 bpm ($p < 0.01$).
Side effects were generally not troublesome and only 3.7% of patients stopped treatment for this reason. The commonest were headache and tiredness.

Introduction

In the last decade interest has increasingly turned to anti-hypertensive agents producing a smoother control of blood pressure, with less postural fluctuation and which are also more acceptable to the patients.

Previous reports have agreed that Labetalol [1,2], commonly used in the treatment of hypertension [3,4], has advantages over other drugs in being relatively free from severe side effects [5,6], though these in some degree are experienced by most patients and some have to stop treatment altogether on this account [7,8]. In many, also, it has not been possible to maintain adequate control over the blood pressure [9].

The aim of this study was to achieve a fairly definitive statement based on a large group of patients studied over a sufficient period of time to draw long-term conclusions.

Patients and Methods

In order to obtain a sufficient number of patients a multi-centre trial was organized. Twenty-eight hospital centres agreed to participate in the study. A total number of 377 outpatients was originally included in the study; however, the paper reports on the results from 277 patients with complete records according to the trial protocol. Criteria for inclusion in the study were: 1) presence of supine diastolic blood pressure ≥ 95 mmHg after 3 consecutive recordings, 2) age between 25 and 75 years, 3) serum creatinine $< 1.5/100$ ml, 4) blood urea < 60 mg/100 ml, 5) absence of conduction disturbances or bradycardia less than 60 bpm, 6) absence of valvular heart disease, 7) no history of congestive heart failure or myocardial infarction in the preceding 6 months. Patients with angina pectoris were also included in the study, while patients suffering from

Table I. *Reasons for withdrawal fron study.*

	No. patients	%
Poor co-operation	83	22.0
Side effects	14	3.7
Poor blood pressure control	3	0.8

asthma, bronchitis and diabetes mellitus were eligible for inclusion at the physician's discretion. Of the 277 patients whose results were analyzed, 155 were male and 122 female. Ages ranged from 32 to 73 years (mean 52.3 ± 10.3 years). On entry, other anti-hypertensive drugs were stopped and after a wash-out period of 7 days Labetalol treatment was started at the dosage of 100 mg b.i.d..

Increments were made as required at each visit. The addition of an oral diuretic to Labetalol was made for purely clinical reasons and, usually, it was prescribed to achieve a better control over blood pressure or in those patients in whom fluid retention occurred. Patients were seen weekly during the first month of therapy and then less frequently, most often fortnightly, when control was established. Blood pressure and heart rate were recorded at each visit after 5 minutes' lying and after 1 minute standing. Because of the large amount of data involved in this study, it became apparent that computer facilities would be necessary. For each patient, therefore, the following data were entered in a computer file: 1) patient number, 2) sex, 3) age, 4) all blood pressure readings and pulse rates at all visits, 5) dosage of Labetalol at each visit, 6) details of the diuretic taken, 7) details of side effects seen, 8) duration of treatment. Finally, patients were classified according to the severity of the disease which was graded according to diastolic

blood pressure as mild (35-100 mmHg), moderate (101-119 mmHg) or severe (> 115 mmHg) hypertension.

Results

All of the patients, investigated along conventional lines, were affected by essential hypertension.

Of the 377 patient record cards originally included, 100 (26.5%) were excluded from the analysis for one reason or another (Table I). Seventy-eight patients were newly diagnosed and the remainder had received previous antihypertensive therapy before the trial. The average duration of the study was 12 weeks. The classification of the patients according to the hypertension severity grading is shown in Table II.

The mean blood pressure and heart rate measured in the whole group at the end of the wash-out period and at the time of the final control are shown in Fig. 1. Labetalol reduced supine systolic blood pressure from 186 ± 20 to 157 ± 21 mmHg (p < 0.01), diastolic from 107 ± 10 to 91 ± 12 mmHg (p < 0.01) and heart rate from 83 ± 10 to 74 ± 9 bpm (p < 0.01). No statistical difference was observed between supine and standing blood pressure values during treatment (Fig. 2). The distribution of systolic and diastolic blood pressure before and after therapy is illustrated in Fig. 3. It can

Table II. *Severity grading.*

Hypertension grade	DBP (mmHg)	No. patients	%
Mild	95 — 100	34	12.3
Moderate	101 — 114	184	66.4
Severe	115	59	21.3

DBP = diastolic blood pressure

134

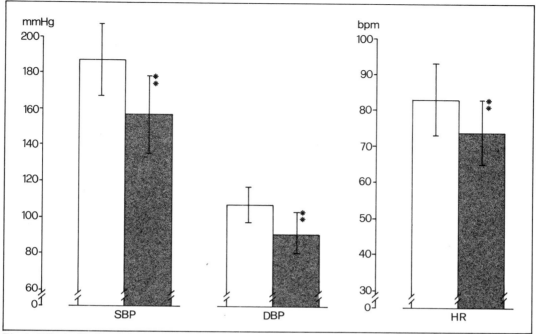

Fig. 1. Effect of Labetalol on systolic blood pressure (SBP), diastolic blood pressure (DBP) and heart rate (HR) in 277 hypertensive patients. Open bars indicate pre-treatment values (Mean ± SD); hatched, after Labetalol. [** p < 0.01 significantly lower than control value].

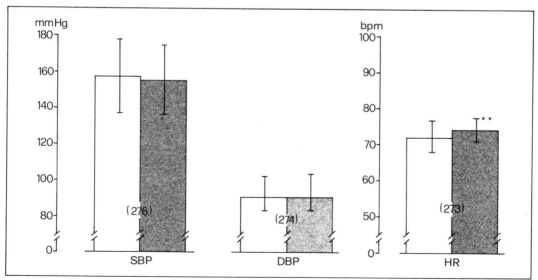

Fig. 2. Comparison between supine and upright arterial pressure and heart rate (Mean ± SD) at the end of the trial. Open bars indicate supine blood pressure; hatched, upright; figures in parentheses are number of patients. [** p < 0.01].

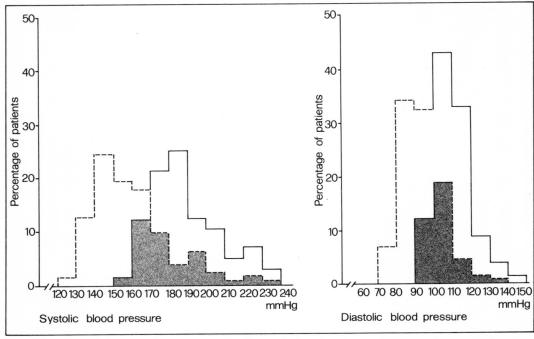

Fig. 3. Systolic and diastolic blood pressure distribution before (continuous line) and while on (dotted line) Labetalol.

be seen from this figure that a significant shift to lower values occurs. Blood pressure and heart rate data obtained in mild, moderate and severe hypertensives are reported in Table III. In all three groups of patients, therapy induced a significant fall in both systolic and diastolic blood pessure, but the decrease in pressure was rather greater in the more severe group, in which the initial pressures were higher.

The result was classified as good if the blood pressure was 160/95 mmHg at the final control and if the patient did not experience any side effects. According to these criteria, the overall results of the trial were that 174 out of 277 patients (62.8%) had a good control. Fig. 4 illustrates the distribution of blood pressure for each patient before and after the therapy. The result, however, was related to the severity of the hypertension, 26/34

Table III. *Mean (± S.D.) supine blood pressure and heart rate before and after Labetalol in patients according to severity of hypertension.*

Hypertension grade	No. patients	SBP (mmHg) before	SBP (mmHg) after	DBP (mmHg) before	DBP (mmHg) after	HR (bpm) before	HR (bpm) after
Mild	34	174±12	151±16	93+5	85+9	82+10	76+9
		($p \diagup 0.01$)		($p < 0.01$)		($p < 0.05$)	
Moderate	184	183±16	156±20	105+4	90+10	82+10	76+9
		($p < 0.01$)		($p < 0.01$)		($p < 0.05$)	
Severe	59	203±22	167±24	122+7	97+13	86+12	74+8
		($p < 0.01$)		($p < 0.01$)		($p < 0.01$)	

SBP = systolic blood pressure; DBP = diastolic blood pressure; HR = heart rate

136

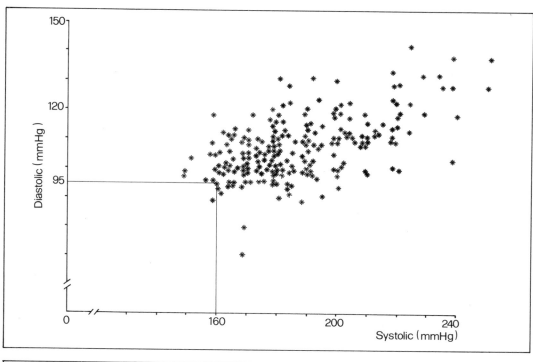

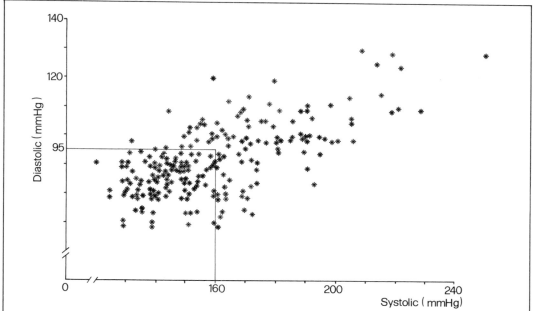

Fig. 4. Distribution of blood pressures before (high panel) and after (low panel) Labetalol (see text).

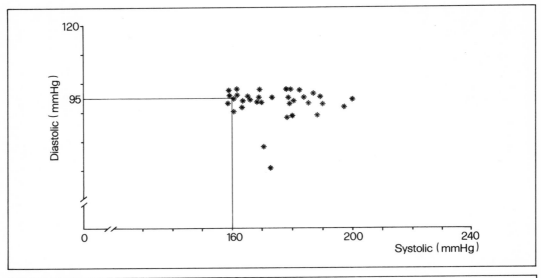

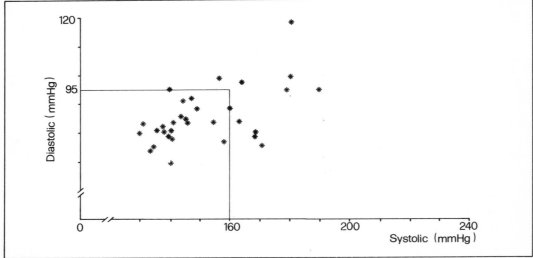

Fig. 5. Distribution of blood pressures (high panel) and after (low panel) Labetalol, in mild hypertension.

(76.5%) of patients with mild hypertension having good control, 120/184 (65.2%) with moderate and 28/59 (47.5%) with severe grade of disease. These data are illustrated in Figs. 5, 6 and 7.

Drug regimen

Patients were classified according to the final therapeutic regimen in 6 different groups, namely:

Group 1: patients treated with Labetalol 100 mg b.i.d.
Group 2: treated with Labetalol 200 mg b.i.d.
Group 3: Labetalol was employed with a treatment schedule different from that of groups 1 and 2
Group 4: treated with Labetalol 100 mg b.i.d. plus a diuretic
Group 5: treated with Labetalol 200 mg b.i.d. plus a diuretic

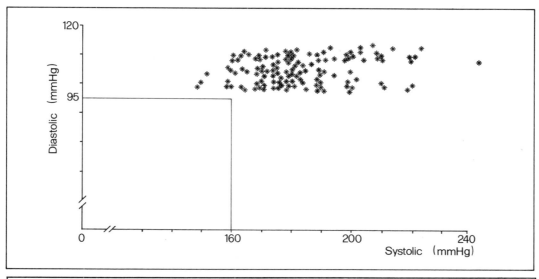

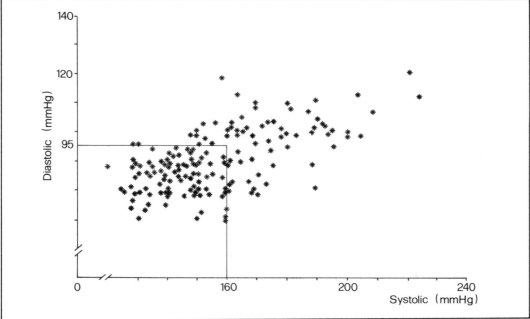

Fig. 6. Distribution of blood pressures before (high panel) and after (low panel) Labetalol, in moderate hypertension.

Group 6: as in group 3 with the addition of a diuretic.

The results obtained in these different groups are shown in Table IV.

From this table it is apparent that a significant reduction in blood pressure was obtained in all treatment groups and that this beneficial effect was achieved in 136 (49.1%) patients using Labetalol twice daily.

Addition of diuretic

An oral diuretic was added to Labetalol in 112 (40.4%) patients. In particular chlorthali-

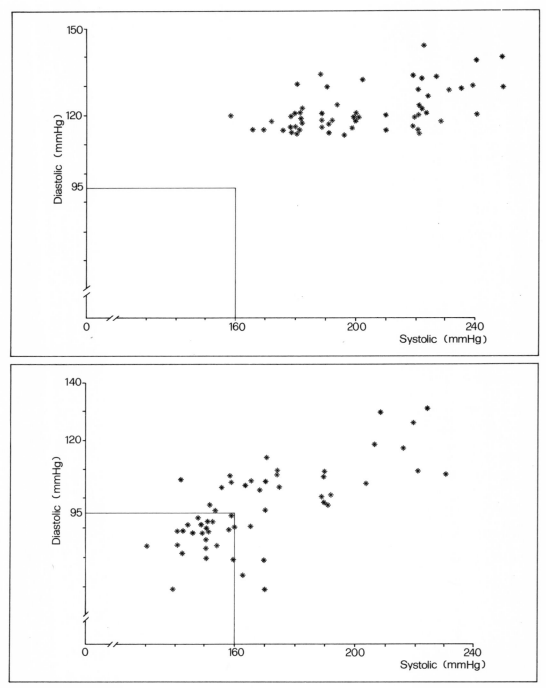

Fig. 7. Distribution of blood pressures before (high panel) and after (low panel) Labetalol, in severe hypertension.

140

Table IV. *Mean (± S.D.) supine blood pressure before (B) and after (A) Labetalol in patients according to treatment grouping. Figures in parentheses are numbers of patients.*

Mild Hypertension

	Group 1 (n=8)	Group 2 (n=1)	Group 3 (n=8)	Group 4 (n=6)	Group 5 (n=0)	Group 6 (n=11)
B	163±5	160	170+8	180±15		182±7
SBP (mmHg)						
A	142±10 $p < 0.01$	145	149±16 $p < 0.01$	152±12 $p < 0.01$		159±15 $p < 0.01$
B	94±2	95	92±5	94±2		92±7
DBP (mmHg)						
A	84±6 $p < 0.01$	85	89±14 $p < 0.01$	83±4 $p < 0.01$		85±10 $p < 0.05$

Moderate Hypertension

	Group 1 (n=48)	Group 2 (n=26)	Group 3 (n=42)	Group 4 (n=10)	Group 5 (n=10)	Group 6 (n=47)
B	179±13	181±17	184±18	185±20	181±15	187±18
SBP (mmHg)						
A	149±16 $p < 0.01$	156±22 $p < 0.01$	155±24 $p < 0.01$	144±14 $p < 0.01$	151±6 $p < 0.01$	167±20 $p < 0.01$
B	105±5	105±4	104±4	105±2	107±3	106±4
DBP (mmHg)						
A	87±9 $p < 0.01$	91±11 $p < 0.01$	90±11 $p < 0.01$	81±7 $p < 0.01$	91±8 $p < 0.01$	93±10 $p < 0.01$
		$p < 0.01$	$p < 0.01$	$p < 0.01$		$p < 0.01$

	Group 1 (n=0)	Group 2 (n=17)	Group 3 (n=15)	Group 4 (n=9)	Group 5 (n=1)	Group 6 (n=17)
B		198±20	206±23	214±25	220	203±23
SBP (mmHg)						
A		164±21 p<0.01	169±24 p<0.01	184±23 p<0.01	170	172±28 p<0.01
B		119±20	123±7	127±8	115	122±8
DBP (mmHg)						
A		93±21 p<0.01	95±12 p<0.01	106±12 p<0.01	80	99±15 p<0.01

done was used in 46 patients, triamterene in 46, furosemide in 10, hydrochlorothiazide in 10. As specified previously, the addition of a diuretic was made for purely clinical reasons and not with a view to making any controlled observations. In 70 patients, however, the diuretic was added without making any other change in treatment or alteration in the dose of Labetalol, and in these patients a controlled comparison is therefore possible between the blood pressure before and after the diuretic (Table V). From this table it is apparent that a further, significant decrease in blood pressure was obtained after the addition of diuretic to Labetalol.

Side effects

Of the 377 patient record cards received, 14 (3.7%) reported side effects severe enough to cause discontinuation of therapy. Table VI presents the 10 most commonly mentioned problems associated with Labetalol and the percentage of such findings. Some patients reported 2 side effects.

Discussion

A number of reports has been published in this country on the treatment of hypertension with Labetalol, but mainly in relatively small series of patients treated for short periods [10-]

Table V. *Fall in blood pressure (70 cases) after addition of diuretic to stabilized dose of Labetalol.*

	After wash-out	After Labetalol	After Labetalol+diuretic
SBP (mmHg)	188±19.4	165±22.7	158±21.2 p < 0.05
DBP (mmHg)	106±11.8	94±12.7	90±12.7 p < 0.05
HR (mmHg)	83±12.8	77± 9.4	76± 8.9 n.s.

Comparison between Labetalol and Labetalol + diuretic blood pressure

142

Table VI. *Percent of adverse reactions to Labetalol requiring cessation of treatment.*

Side effects	%
1. Headache	2.1
2. Tiredness	2.1
3. Somnolence	1.06
4. Sexual disturbance	0.9
5. Dyspnea	0.8
6. Palpitations	0.8
7. Skin rash	0.5
8. Orthostatic hypertension	0.5
9. Nasal congestion	0.2
10. Vivid dreams	0.2
11. Others	1.6

[12]. This study reports the clinical experience of 28 hospital centres on 377 hypertensive patients treated with Labetalol during an average period of 12 weeks.

The results of this large, multi-centre, open study indicate that Labetalol is an effective long-term agent for lowering blood pressure in all grades of hypertension, with a very desirable type of blood pressure control, with easily identifiable and reversible side effects.

Most beta-blockers have been successfully employed in the treatment of hypertension; Labetalol combines beta-adrenoceptor with alpha-adrenoceptor blocking properties [13, 14], thus allowing a hypotensive effect with a more favourable hemodynamic profile than with beta-adrenoceptor blockade alone [15, 16]. This study confirms the good balance between alpha- and beta-adrenoceptor antagonism achieved by Labetalol. Actually, although the therapy reduced the pulse rate, the mean supine pulse rate of 74 bpm was rather higher than mean values reported during treatment with beta-blockers [17-19]. Moreover, no change between supine and standing blood pressure was observed at the end of the trial.

A substantial decrease in blood pressure occurred when Labetalol was given alone. The addition of an oral diuretic was made for purely clinical reasons in 112 subjects. It was prescribed to achieve a better control over blood pressure or in those patients in whom fluid retention occurred. In 70 patients, however, the diuretic was added without making any other change in the dose of Labetalol, and a controlled comparison is therefore possible between the blood pressures before and after the diuretic. An appreciable, additional fall in blood pressure was observed in these patients when the diuretic was added to Labetalol.

There have been attempts to reduce the number of daily doses in beta-adrenoceptor blocking therapy while maintaining the anti-hypertensive effects. This is an aspect which is of great practical interest. The difficulties of keeping the patient on regular therapy in the treatment of hypertension are documented in many studies [20, 21]. One way of overcoming this problem may be to make administration of the drug concerned as simple as possible, e.g. twice or perhaps even once daily. Actually, there is evidence to suggest that medication errors and drug defaulting are proportional to the number of doses taken each day [22]. In this study Labetalol was given twice daily in 136 patients (49%) and, as illustrated in Table IV, a significant fall in blood pressure was obtained in all treatment groups (Groups 1, 2, 4, 5).

Therapy with Labetalol, as in the case of all anti-hypertensive drugs, is associated with certain unpleasant side effects. However, two rather disabling problems common to all drugs which block sympathetic activity, i.e. orthostatic hypotension and sexual dysfunction, do not occur as frequently with this drug as with guanethidine or methyldopa. Table VI presents side effects which required cessation of therapy in 14 patients. Orthostatic hypotension was mentioned with a frequency of 0.5%, and sexual disturbances were rare (0.9%).

The other adverse reactions were troublesome but not of major consequence. In those patients, in whom the presence of side effects did not require discontinuation of the treatment, the adverse reactions were generally mild and usually transient in nature.

In conclusion, the results of this multi-centre, open study confirm the findings of earlier investigations carried out in small numbers of patients and show that Labetalol is an effective and well tolerated drug for treating hypertension.

References

1. Brittain R.T., Levy G.P.: A review of the animal pharmacology of labetalol, a combined α- and β-adrenoceptor blocking drug. *Br. J. Clin. Pharmacol.* 3, 681, 1976.
2. Richards D.A.: Pharmacological effects of labetalol in man. *Br. J. Clin. Pharmacol.* 3, 721, 1976.
3. Prichard B.N.C., Boakes A.J., Hernandez R.: Long-term treatment of hypertension with labetalol. *Br. J. Clin. Phamarcol.* 8, 171S, 1979.
4. Simpson F.O., Bailey R.R., Campbell D.G., Dickson D.S.P., Kiddle G.B., Lewis G.R.J., Logan R., Harrison R.B., Poole A.P., Turner A.S., Waal-Manning H.J., Wood A.J.: A multicentre open trial of labetalol in New Zealand. *Br. J. Clin. Pharmacol.* 8, 179S, 1979.
5. Kane J., Gregg I., Stephens M.D.B.: A long-term study of Labetalol in general practice. *Br. J. Clin. Pharmacol.* 8, 167S, 1979.
6. Richards D.A., Jackson J.L.: Post-clinical surveillance of labetalol. In: Fletchen E. (ed.): *Drug symposium on labetalol*, Florence, April 1979, p. 105.
7. Pugsley D.J., Armstrong B.K., Nassim M.A., Beilin L.J.: Controlled comparison of labetalol and propranolol in the management of severe hypertension. *Br. J. Clin. Pharmacol.* 3, 777, 1976.
8. Prichard B.N.C., Boakes A.J.: Labetalol in long-term treatment of hypertension. *Br. J. Clin. Pharmacol.* 3, 743, 1976.
9. Alves I., Gouveia A., De Andrade N., Ribeiro A., Carrageta M.: Effect of labetalol administered once in essential hypertension. In: Fletcher E. (ed.): *Drug symposium on labetalol*, Florence, April 1979, p. 129.
10. Danti G. et al.: The effectiveness of long-term treatment of mild to severe hypertension with labetalol. *Clin. Terap.* 93, 169, 1980.
11. Pedrazzi F., Bommartini F.: Possibilities and limitations of the use of labetalol in the treatment of hypertension in the elderly. *G. Gerontol* 28, 113, 1980.
12. Rossi A., Ziacchi V., Lomanto B.: A clinical evaluation of labetalol in essential hypertension. Effects of chronic treatment in conditions of rest and stress. *Minerva Cardioangiol.* 28, 637, 1980.
13. Richards D.A., Prichard B.N.C.: Clinical pharmacology of labetalol. *Br. J. Clin. Pharmacol.* 8, 89S, 1979.
14. Brittain R.T.: The pharmacology of labetalol. In: Fletcher, E. (ed.): *Drug symposium on labetalol*, Florence, April 1979, pag. 9.
15. Metha J., Cohn J.N.: Haemodynamic effects of labetalol, an alpha and beta-adrenergic blocking agent, in hypertensive subjects. *Circulation* 55, 370, 1977.
16. Koch G.: Cardiovascular dynamics after acute and long-term alpha and beta-adrenoceptor blockade at rest, supine and standing. *Br. J. Clin. Phamarcol.* 3 (Suppl. 3), 729, 1976.
17. Lund-Johansen P., Ohm O.S.: Hemodynamic long-term effects of metoprolol at rest and during exercise in essential hypertension. *Br. J. Clin. Pharmacol.* 3, 147, 1977.
18. Wilcox R.G.: Randomized study of six beta-blockers and a thiazide diuretic in essential hypertension. *Br. Med. J.* 2, 383, 1978.
19. Douglas-Jones A.P., Cruickshank J.M.: Once-daily dosing with atenolol in patients with mild or moderate hypertension. *Br. Med. J.* 1, 990, 1976.
20. Caldwell J.R., Cobb S., Dowling M.D., De Jong D.: The drop-out problem in antihypertensive treatment. *J. Chron, Dis.* 22, 579, 1970.
21. Frithz J., Hood B., Hansson L, Bjork S.: Cerebrovascular lesions. Active antihypertensive treatment and the present situation. *Acta Med. Scand.* 196, 35, 1974.
22. Molahy B.: The effect of instruction and labelling on the number of medication errors made by patients at home. *Am. J. Hosp. Pharm.* 23, 283, 1966.

Hypertension, recent advances and research
edited by M. Condorelli, A. Zanchetti
Cortina International, Verona 1982

Infusion treatment with Labetalol in acute hypertensive states

F. SORRENTINO, S. SIGNORELLI, G.M. ANDREOZZI

2nd Institute of Special Pathological Medicine and Clinical Methodology, University of Catania, Italy

Key words. Labetalol i.v.; Infusion Treatment; Acute Hypertension; Hypertensive Crises; Side Effects; Rest Flow; Peak Flow; Venous Occlusion Plethysmography; Transient Cerebral Ischaemic Attacks; Beta-blocking Effect; Alpha-blocking Effect.

Summary. Labetalol would appear to possess many properties which justify its inclusion in the category of those drugs useful for the treatment of hypertensive crises.

Our experience with Labetalol relates to the 50-75 mg. bolus administration of the drug in 12 cases of hypertension, not all of which, however, could be considered emergency cases.

In 8 of these patients the bolus was followed by continuous 3-hour infusion with progressive doses of the drug: 1 mg/kg b.w. at hour 1, 2 mg/kg b.w. at hour 2, and 4 mg/kg b.w. at hour 3.

In all patients, both in response to the bolus injection and the infusion, there was a reduction in blood pressure as regards both maximum and minimum values.

All patients showed a modest reduction in Heart Rate.

At no time did we encounter side effects of such a nature as to induce us to suspend the infusion.

In addition, we studied the Rest Flow and Peak Flow (i.e. after ischaemia) in the muscle region of the calf using infinite-time-constant venous-occlusion plethysmography.

The muscle flow behaviour in the region explored was similar to that documented in our previous research work on beta-blocker drugs. This would lead us to presume that in this region, too, the beta-blocking effect of Labetalol is greater than its alpha-blocking effect.

In certain situations, regardless of the absolute levels reached, the sudden rise in BP may cause irreparable damage to the human body. This occurs when there is another associated pathological condition present, such as ischaemic heart disease, acute left ventricular insufficiency, dessicative aneurysm of the aorta or transient cerebral ischaemic attacks. Such conditions generally require immediate intervention.

Today there are many drugs capable of reducing BP speedily and efficiently and, as the critical hypertensive state is maintained - from the pathophysiological point of view - by peripheral resistances, these drugs act by lowering the peripheral resistances; in other words, they are vasodilatory.

Regrettably, the use of such drugs may be limited by their side effects; for example, their reflex effects on the heart (tachycardia, increased stroke volume, greater oxygen consumption, etc.) and the increased intravascular volume.

The continuous search for new substances which are effective against hypertension and at the same time low in side effects is therefore fully justified.

The ideal drug should have the following properties: easy administration, prompt and efficacious effect and the ability to reduce vascular resistance - all with no or limited side effects

We therefore decided to carry out a study on the use of Labetalol in cases of acute hypertension, given that - as this congress has amply illustrated - Labetalol possesses the necessary properties and action suitable for such cases.

Methods

Eighteen male patients aged between 48 and 65 years participated in the study. All were suffering from 2nd degree hypertension, with frequent paroxysmal rises in blood pressure.

The increase in BP was accompanied in 6 patients by severe headache; in 8 patients the rise in BP called for urgent therapy of associated ischaemic heart disease, and in 4 it was accompanied by transient cerebral ischaemia (TIA).

In 6 patients, four with coronary disorders and two with transient cerebral ischaemia, blood pressure exceeded 240 mm/Hg and was accompanied by angina and TIA symptoms.

These patients received fast 2-minute intravenous administration of Labetalol at the rate of 1 mg/kg of body weight. The patients were also found to have less serious hypertensive conditions but were treated nonetheless on account of their associated pathology.

All patients, including the 12 whose BP did not reach such high levels, were first given a fast intravenous dose of the drug at the rate of 1 mg/kg of body weight, and then were administered increasing doses by slow infusion (1 mg/kg in the first hour, 2 mg/kg in the second hour, 4 mg/kg in the third hour). Heart rate and systolic and diastolic BP were monitored, taking special care to note the appearance of possible side effects.

Muscle flow was assessed in all patients, during rest and after ischaemia, in the region of the calf by means of infinite-time-constant venous occlusion plethysmography. This method may be subject to criticism with regard to the absolute flow values, but it is extremely useful for a pharmacodynamic study.

For details regarding the recording techniques, we refer readers to our previous publications.

Results

None of our patients experienced any unpleasant side effects.

In the 6 patients with very high BP the fast "bolus" administration of the drug brought about a rapid reduction in BP within 5 to 15 minutes: systolic pressure was reduced from mean values of 225 mmHg to 185 mmHg, whilst diastolic pressure was reduced from 125 mmHg to 105 mmHg.

The lowering of BP in coronary disease patients was accompanied by a diminution in the clinical symptoms; the patients with TIA were given vasoactive drugs immediately after the administration of Labetalol.

Fig. 1 shows the behaviour of blood pressure 18 minutes after the fast "bolus" administration of Labetalol at the dose of 1mg/kg of

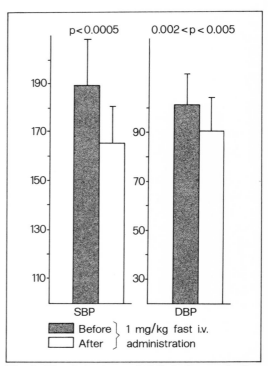

Fig. 1. The behaviour of B.P. before and after administration of Labetalol (i.v.).

body weight. The reduction in the maximum and minimum pressures is highly significant.

Fig. 2 shows the effect on systolic and diastolic BP, the flow during rest and after ischaemia, and on HR after intravenous Labetalol administration. Flow during rest does not vary

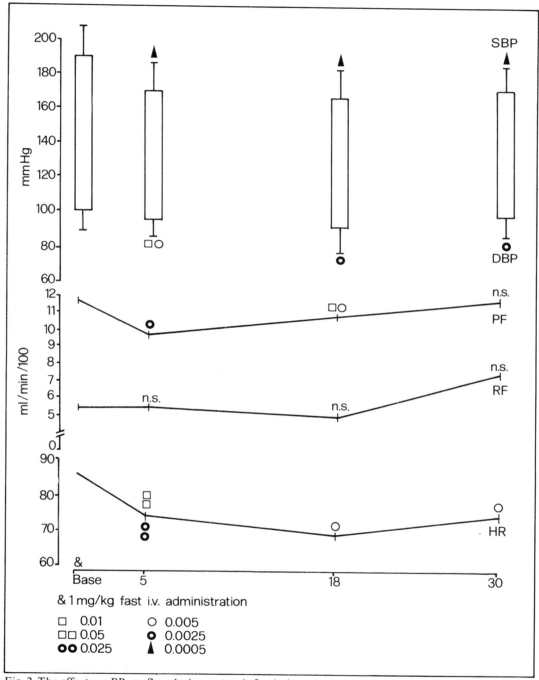

Fig. 2. The effects on BP, on flow during rest and after ischaemia, and on HR after Labetalol administration (1 mg/kg i.v.).

significantly, but the peak flow shows significant variations after 5 and 18 minutes. HR, on the other hand, is considerably reduced, perhaps also as compared to the very high starting values.

According to these results, and as other authors have already confirmed, when Labetalol is administerd by bolus its beta-blocking action is more marked than its alpha-blocking action.

But if we compare behaviour after the administration of a cardioselective beta-blocking drug like Metoprolol, we find that BP reductions are smaller and concern especially the maximum values (Fig. 3); we also find that muscle flow during rest and after ischaemia is reduced, whereas with Labetalol it remains unaltered.

In our opinion this would indicate that the alpha-blocking effect is not absent but merely overshadowed by the predominant beta-blocking effects.

But this could also be due to the fact that the area we examined does not generally have a high content of alpha-receptors, which are predominantly found at skin vessel level.

Looking at the results of the infusion (Fig. 4), we can see that blood pressure begins to

descend significantly after 30 minutes and continues to decrease more and more as the drug concentration increases.

Heart rate, not shown on the graph, undergoes no significant alteration.

Flow in the rest position increases after about 120 minutes while peak flow increases significantly after 90 and 180 minutes. This behaviour might be explained by the observations of other authors, namely that beta-blocking effects are more evident with smaller doses, whilst alpha-blocking effects predominate with greater doses.

Remarks

In conclusion we may say that Labetalol administered intravenously determines a significant and rapid fall in BP, both systolic and diastolic.

Heart rate decreases if the drug is administered via bolus but does not change if administered by infusion.

Muscle flow during rest and post-ischaemic muscle flow remain unchanged after fast intravenous administration. Strano's group noted the same behaviour, i.e. no modifications in the rheographic indices following the intravenous administration of Labetalol. During infusion at higher doses, flow increase is observed.

The results obtained regarding muscle flow might give rise to doubts as to the alpha-blocking vasodilatory effect of the drug; but we believe this situation can be explained as follows:

1) with bolus administration, the beta effects are more obvious, but the alpha effects are nonetheless present, for there is no modification in flow behaviour after Labetalol whereas after the administration of a beta-blocking drug, albeit cardioselective, flow is seen to decrease;

2) the higher the dose the more evident the increase;

3) the absence of noticeable effects on flow during rest may also be explained by the relative scarcity of alpha-receptors in the musculoskeletal region, whereas they would be more abundant at skin vessel level.

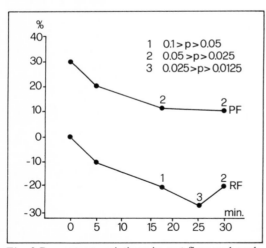

Fig. 3 Percentage variations in rest flow and peak flow induced by the i.v. administration of 5 mg of metoprolol (10 cases). (R.F. = Rest Flow; nean basal value assumed as zero) (P.F. = Peak Flow; expressed as % increment in relation to instantaneous R.F.).

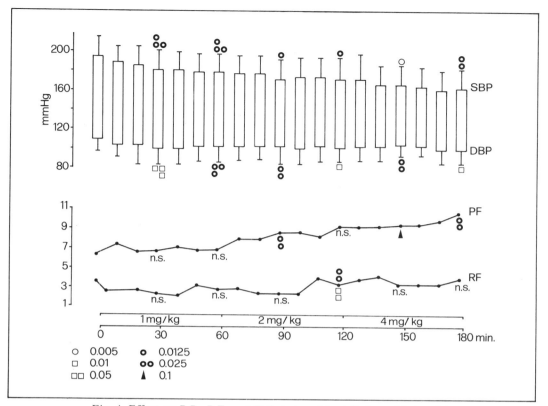

Fig. 4. Effect on B.P., P.F. and R.F. induced by infusion of Labetalol.

These considerations should suffice, in our opinion, to dispel all doubts about the alpha-blocking effects of Labetalol.

Another important fact revealed by our study is the absence of side effects.

The effects we have illustrated therefore make us inclined to support the use of this drug for the therapy of acute hypertension accompanied by ischaemic heart conditions and transient cerebral ischaemic attacks.

We have restricted ourselves to these recommendations because these arise directly from our analysis, but we feel certain that the drug could be usefully employed in other cases of acute hypertension such as pheochromocytoma and the clonidine withdrawal crises.

We are not, however, convinced that the drug should be used in hypertensive crises where there is left ventricular insufficiency.

References

1. Andersson O., Goran B., Lennart H.: Anti-hypertensive action, time of onset and effects on carbohydrate metabolism of labetalol. *Br. J. Clin. Pharmacol.* 757-761, 1976.

2. Agabiti Rosei E., Brown J.J., Lever A.F., Robertson J.I.S., Trust P.: Treatment of pheochromocytoma and clonidine withdrawal hypertension with labetalol. *Br. J. Pharmacol.* 809-815, 1976.

3. Bolli P., Hendrika J., Wood A.J., Simpson F.C.: Experience with labetalol in hypertension. *Br. J. Pharmacol.* 765-771, 1976.

4. Edwards R.C., Raffery E.B.: Haemodynamic effects of long-term oral labetalol. *Br. J. Pharmacol.* 733-736, 1976.

5. Koch G.: Combined alpha and beta-adrenoceptor blockade with oral labetalol in hypertensive patients with reference to haemodynamic effects at rest and during exercise. *Br. J. Pharmacol.* 729-732, 1976.

6. Koch G.: Acute haemodynamic effects of an alpha and beta-receptor blocking agent (AH 5158) on the systemic and pulmonary circulation at rest and during

exercise in hypertensive patients. *Amer. Heart J.* 93, 5, 1977.

7. Jockes A.M., Thompson F.D.: Acute haemodynamic effects of labetalol and its subsequent use as an oral hypotensive agent. *Br. J. Pharmacol.* 789-793, 1976.

8. Moulds R.F., Jaureing R.A., Hobson J.D., Shaw J.: Effects of the beta-receptor antagonist propranolol, oxprenolol and labetalol on human vascular smooth-muscle contraction. *Clin. Sci. Mol. Med.* 55, 235-240, 1978.

9. Mancia G., Ferrari A., Gregorini L., Ferrari M., Bianchini C., Terzoli L., Leonetti G., Zanchetti A.: Effetti della prazosina sulla emodinamica basale e sul controllo nervoso della circolazione nel paziente iperteso. *Farmaci*, Suppl. n. 2, 12, 78.

10. Mehta J., Cohn J.N.: Haemodynamic effects of labetalol, an alpha and beta-adrenergic blocking agent, in hypertensive subjects. *Circulation* 55, 2, 1977.

11. Pearson R.M., Havard C.W.: Intravenous labetalol in hypertensive patients given by fast and slow injection. *Br. J. Pharmacol.* 5, 401-405, 1978.

12. Phillips L.A.: Labetalol: a clinical review. *J. Pharmacol.* 1, 35, 1977.

13. Richards D.A., Prichard B.N., Boakes A.J., Tuckman J., Knight E.: Pharmacological basis for antihypertensive effects of intravenous labetalol. *Brit. Heart J.* 39, 99-106, 1977.

14. Richards D.A., Woodings E.P., Stephens B., Macono-chie J.G.: The effects of oral AH 5158, a combined alpha and beta-adrenoceptor antagonist, in healthy volunteers. *Brit. J. Clin. Pharmacol.* 1, 505-510, 1974.

15. Richards D.A.: Pharmacological effects of labetalol in man. *Brit. J. Clin. Pharmacol.* 721-723, 1976.

16. Richards D.A., Maconochie J.G., Bland R.E., Hopkins R., Woodings E.P. Martin L.E.: Relationship between plasma concentrations and pharmacological effects of labetalol. *Europ. J. Clin. Pharmacol.* 11, 85-90, 1977.

17. Ronne J.O. Rasmussen G.S., Andersen N., Bowal J., Andersson E.: Acute effect of intravenous labetalol treatment of systemic arterial hypertension. *Br. J. Clin. Pharmacol.* 805-808, 1976.

18. Strano A., Novo S., Davì G., Pinto A., Riolo F.: Comportamento dei valori tensivi arteriosi e della reattività vascolare a riposo e dopo sforzo, in soggetti ipertesi trattati con labetalolo per via endovenosa. pp. 93-102. In: *Atti Conv. Int. Ipertensione: Nuove prospettive terapeutiche.* Venezia, 18-20 maggio 1978. Glaxo Italia 1978, 269.

19. Trust P.M., Rosei E.A., Brown J.J., Fraser R., Lever A.F. Morton J.J., Robertson J.I.: Effects of blood pressure, angiotensin II and aldosterone concentrations during treatment of severe hypertension with intravenous labetalol. Comparison with propranolol. *Br. J. Clin. Pharmacol.* 799-803, 1976.

Index

PRINTED IN ITALY
BY "BERTONCELLO ARTIGRAFICHE"
CITTADELLA (PADOVA).
SEPTEMBER 1982.